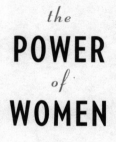

the
POWER
of
WOMEN

the

POWER

of

WOMEN

A DOCTOR'S JOURNEY OF
HOPE AND HEALING

DR. DENIS MUKWEGE

FLATIRON
BOOKS
NEW YORK

The names of my patients have been changed in most cases, with the exception being those who have waived their right to anonymity or who are identified in the text as public campaigners.

THE POWER OF WOMEN. Copyright © 2021 by Denis Mukwege. All rights reserved. Printed in the United States of America. For information, address Flatiron Books, 120 Broadway, New York, NY 10271.

www.flatironbooks.com

Map courtesy of the UN Office for the Coordination of Humanitarian Affairs

Design by Donna Sinisgalli Noetzel

Library of Congress Cataloging-in-Publication Data

Names: Mukwege, Denis, author.
Title: The power of women : a doctor's journey of hope and healing / Dr. Denis Mukwege.
Description: First edition. | New York : Flatiron Books, 2021. | Includes bibliographical references and index.
Identifiers: LCCN 2021026474 | ISBN 9781250769190 (hardcover) | ISBN 9781250769268 (ebook)
Subjects: LCSH: Mukwege, Denis. | Physicians—Congo (Democratic Republic) | Women—Violence against—Africa. | Sexual abuse victims—Africa. | Rape victims—Africa. | Women and war—Africa. | Resilience (Personality trait)—Africa. | Women—Africa—Social conditions.
Classification: LCC HV6569.C75 M843 2021 | DDC 610.82096—dc23
LC record available at https://lccn.loc.gov/2021026474

Our books may be purchased in bulk for promotional, educational, or business use. Please contact your local bookseller or the Macmillan Corporate and Premium Sales Department at 1-800-221-7945, extension 5442, or by email at MacmillanSpecialMarkets@macmillan.com.

First Edition: 2021

10 9 8 7 6 5 4 3 2 1

To my mother, my wife, my daughters, and my sisters.

To all the victims of sexual violence.

CONTENTS

Map   *ix*

Introduction   *xi*

1. Maternal Courage   1

2. A Women's Health Crisis   23

3. Crisis and Resilience   44

4. Pain and Power   74

5. In His Words   101

6. Speaking Out   127

7. Fighting for Justice   156

8. Recognition and Remembrance   187

9. Men and Masculinity   212

10. Leadership   236

Conclusion   263

Acknowledgments   279

Notes   281

Index   289

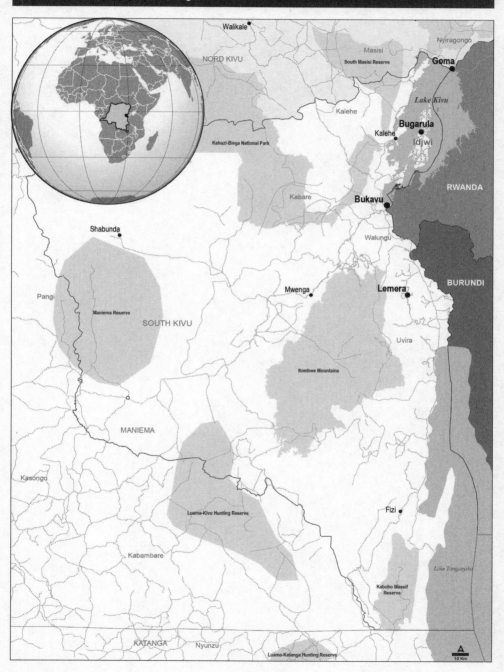

INTRODUCTION

It's unusual for a man to campaign for women's rights. I know this. I've sensed it during conversations with friends, at social gatherings, and occasionally in professional meetings. I've noted the uncomprehending looks and quizzical expressions. Every once in a while, I encounter hostility, whether open or implied. Some find my choices suspicious or even threatening.

I remember dinner parties earlier in my career, in Congo and in Europe, when my turn would come to talk about my work. I would explain that I was a gynecologist who ran a hospital specializing in treating injuries caused by rape. And that I campaigned for women's rights. The table would fall quiet afterward, or someone would ask a polite follow-up question and then switch the subject of the conversation.

In the moments of awkward silence, I could sense sympathy in the eyes of other guests, too: what terrible work, and how I must struggle with my identity, I imagined them thinking. I adopted a strategy of emphasizing how I was also happily married and had children, as if this would make me seem more "normal" or easier to relate to.

Upon arriving back home afterward, I'd lie on my bed or in my hotel room, resenting that I'd felt the need to justify myself. This will be familiar to anyone who has felt the sting of not quite "fitting in" for reasons of origin, identity, or experience.

At other times, people around me would be more blunt. I remember a conversation with an old friend of mine, a classmate from school who became a politician in my province. His words still stick in my mind all these years later. "I feel like since you've been working on sexual violence, you've started thinking like a woman," he once told me. Though this should have been a compliment, it was not intended as such.

I recall the flush of reassurance and kinship I felt when I first discovered the writings and work of Stephen Lewis, a Canadian diplomat and activist who has been a tireless campaigner for AIDS/HIV victims in Africa and women's rights generally. Stephen made me realize that there were other men who thought as I did. I now count him as a dear friend.

You might think that I no longer have to explain my choices after two decades of caring for and treating survivors of sexual violence, but you'd be wrong. And it's not only men who find it hard to understand.

A few years ago, I attended a meeting with a senior figure at the United Nations in New York City. She agreed to receive me along with fellow campaigners working on women's rights and conflict resolution in my country, the Democratic Republic of the Congo. We made our way to the upper floors of her building and were shown to her office, with its large meeting table and extraordinary views over the East River to Queens and Brooklyn beyond.

I was caught off guard by an aggressive interrogation. "Why are you here talking about women's rights in Congo, rather than Congolese women?" our host snapped at me from her place at the table. "Aren't there Congolese women who can speak for themselves?"

The very reason I was there was to request that the UN support initiatives to promote women's voices in Congo. My hospital and foundation have helped survivors find strength in unity and supported individuals in developing their public-speaking and advocacy skills. You will meet many of these inspiring women in this book.

One might argue that the UN official was right to be on her guard against a man seeking to claim a platform for himself that belonged to women. That is a legitimate issue and one that I am always happy to address.

For my own part, whenever I have found myself questioned, at dinner parties or in UN offices, I return to my core convictions. I defend women because they are my equals—because women's rights are human rights, and I am outraged by the violence inflicted on my fellow humans. We must fight for women collectively.

My role has always been to amplify the voices of others whose marginalization denies them opportunities to tell their stories. I stand at their side, never in front.

As you will read, I am in many ways an accidental feminist and campaigner. There was nothing inevitable about my path in life. I set out to become a physician, which was already a lofty ambition for a child born in a shack at a time when Congo was a Belgian colony. But my life has been shaped by events beyond my control, above all the wars since 1996 that have ravaged Congo, and women in particular, under the mostly indifferent gaze of the rest of the world.

Circumstances forced me to become a specialist in treating rape injuries. The stories of the patients I encountered and treated drove me to join a much larger fight against the injustices and cruelties suffered by women. Recognition of my grassroots campaigning has led me to address you in these pages.

My life is intertwined with my war-torn country. Its tumultuous history of exploitation and conflict cries out for much wider understanding. The unrest of the last twenty-five years, the deadliest conflict since World War II, with more than five million dead or missing, has been allowed to metastasize without resolution since 1996. I write of the tragedy of Congo in hopes of encouraging politicians in the West and elsewhere to engage with it, to work toward the peace and justice so desperately desired by the Congolese people. But I have not written an autobiography and still less a book that seeks to explain Congo's wars in full.

This book is a tribute to the power of all women, and in particular those who have raised, educated, and inspired me. As you will see in chapter 1, I start at the very beginning, with the woman who faced down danger and uncertainty to deliver me—and was then called on just days later to save me from illness. The endurance and bravery my mother displayed at my birth was matched only by her lifelong commitment to me and all of her children. She shaped the attitudes of the young man I became, and she also pushed me, occasionally using the benevolent arts of maternal manipulation, to pursue my dreams of becoming a doctor. She was my first hero.

Joining my mother in these pages are many others who have moved me with their courage and kindness, their resilience and energy. They are activists, lawyers, or academics, but they are also patients of mine or the survivors of sexual violence I have met during my years of work in Congo and my travels to Korea, Kosovo, Iraq, Colombia, or the United States, among other places.

The backdrop might appear bleak, for the lives of many women in this book have, like my own, been overshadowed by violence. But these women are each a light and an inspiration, demonstrating how the best instincts of humanity—to love, to share, to protect others—can triumph in the worst-possible circumstances. They are the reason I have persevered for so long. They are the reason I have never lost my faith and sanity even when my work grappling with the consequences of wickedness risked overwhelming me.

Before going further, I want to explain the language I have chosen to use. This is a tricky area because the terms and labels we use to describe people who have experienced sexual violence are significant yet always imperfect. You will notice that I deploy "patient," "victim," and "survivor" to describe many of the women in this book.

"Patient" is the most neutral and requires little explanation. Everyone I have treated is a patient.

The word "victim" is more troublesome because it is associated with weakness and tends to inspire pity. It can make the subject sound passive or fragile and is also the opposite of the word "victor," with which it shares the same Latin root.

"Survivor" has become popular to describe everyone who has experienced sexual violence. It is more active, spirited, and dynamic. Yet some feminist writers find this term problematic, too, seeing it as equating rape with a traumatic, life-altering event such as an attempted murder or a plane crash. It can also reinforce expectations that a woman has overcome the experience and her injuries when it may not feel that way to her.

I try to use these different labels in very specific ways and whenever they feel most appropriate. Many of my patients arrive as victims, which is how they see themselves. They have been subjected to the most serious forms of sexual assault and often attempted murder. In those early instants, no other word seems appropriate for women who have been battered, gang-raped, shot, mutilated, or starved.

But using their own inner strength, we aim to transform them into survivors, in the most accurate sense of that word. We want them to feel that they have overcome their ordeals. Their attackers might have attempted to take their life or destroy their dignity, but we do everything in our power to restore them physically and mentally. If a woman enters feeling like a victim, we want her to leave with the confidence of a survivor. This process is the very essence of our work at Panzi Hospital, which I founded in 1999.

I have spent years talking to survivors. They have shown great trust in me by confiding intimate details about their experiences, their feelings, their fears and hopes. It has often been distressing work, but what drives me as an activist is the belief that something positive can result from all this hardship: that I might contribute, on the survivors' behalf, to making the world a safer place for women.

The latter chapters of the book lay out ways to combat violence against women, drawn from my perspective as a doctor who has worked in a conflict zone and as an activist who has traveled widely to listen to women around the world. I encourage you throughout to see Congo, still sometimes referred to as the "rape capital of the world," as a window onto the extreme end of the global scourge of sexual violence. This is a universal problem that occurs in homes and in businesses, on battlefields and in public spaces, all across the world.

My experience has taught me that the root causes of sexual violence, and its consequences, are the same everywhere. As always, the differences between us in terms of race, nationality, language, and culture are far less significant than what we have in common.

The fight against sexual violence begins with women and men speaking out. One in three women worldwide has experienced either physical or sexual violence at some point in her life, according to UN Women. Nearly one in five women in the United States has experienced completed or attempted rape during her lifetime, according to the Centers for Disease Control and Prevention. We cannot fight this without publicly acknowledging the sheer pervasiveness of the problem.

Fortunately, women are rending the veil of silence around this issue in ever greater numbers, thanks to decades of work from feminist groups and recently the groundbreaking #MeToo movement.

Yet many of them are being let down by the criminal justice system. Judging by the extraordinarily infrequent successful prosecutions of rapists, even in countries with well-funded and corruption-free legal systems, rape remains effectively decriminalized across the world. In conflict zones, soldiers use rape as a weapon of war and have even less reason to fear ending up in prison.

Progress has been made, but mostly on paper through stronger domestic laws or international legislation designed to protect women during conflicts. Women everywhere still fear going to the police to lodge a rape complaint or consider it a waste of time. I will discuss ways for law enforcement and policy makers to provide women with reassurance and to deter rapists in the first place.

While this is primarily a book about women, it is not only for women. It is my fervent hope that people of all genders will read it and educate themselves. We need more active participants in the struggle for gender equality. Men should not fear incomprehension or feel the need to justify themselves, as I once did, when they step up to support their sisters, daughters, wives, mothers, friends, and fellow human beings.

Women cannot solve the problem of sexual violence on their own; men must be part of the solution.

Men continue to retain an overwhelming grip on political power in all countries, not just through the presidencies, prime ministers' offices, and parliaments of the world that set our laws. Their influence extends to the apex of religious bodies and to community-level organizations that often have a more powerful influence on personal behavior and attitudes than distant national leaders.

To reduce sexual violence, we need action and commitment all the way down the pyramid of power in our societies, from the top to the very bottom. As well as looking at the roles of leaders, I will devote one of the latter chapters to the importance of what I call "positive masculinity" and parenting. It will explain how we must educate boys differently to avoid perpetuating the destructive cycle of gender relations that relegates women to second-class citizens.

My work is long term and sometimes frustratingly slow. As a doctor, I can examine a patient, diagnose the source of the problem, and then work to solve it through treatment or surgery. As a campaigner, I face a struggle to change minds, attitudes, and behaviors. It is a battle not with disease or anatomical failure but with far more stubborn adversaries: discrimination, ignorance, and indifference.

Satisfaction comes in rare but uplifting moments of progress. Over the decade and a half of my activism, these have added up to significant gains in our collective understanding of sexual violence.

My hope is that this book helps further one of the greatest causes of the modern era: the campaign for women's rights. Together we can make the twenty-first century a more equal, fairer, and safer century for all of humanity.

1

MATERNAL COURAGE

*M*y mother had endured and triumphed twice before, for the births of my two older sisters. When the contractions gripped her body this third time, for me, she was familiar with the feeling but no less apprehensive. As she paced our family home, the pain and the phases of labor seemed to be following their usual pattern, but the outcome was anything but certain. Might fate, with all of its indifferent cruelty, inflict the suffering of fetal dystocia, the various birth complications that I would later learn by heart?

If so, there was little hope. My mother was alone, save for a neighbor who had joined her when her waters broke. My sisters had been sent to friends' homes. My father was away studying in the south of the province.

The neighbor mouthed words of support and encouragement. She walked in step with my mother when she took to her feet and mopped her brow when she lay down. She readied a razor blade for the final act of delivery, but she brought no medical expertise.

It was 1955. Our house was a typical homestead for poor Black families of the era: flimsy wood and brick walls in a rough rectangular shape, with metal sheeting slung over the top to protect us from the tropical rains that fall throughout the year in Congo. It was the most basic of human constructions, still found today wherever families must shelter with little means.

Comprised of a single room, it had been knocked together rapidly next to others accommodating Congolese families who had come to seek a new life in Bukavu. Once a small fishing village on the banks of Lake Kivu, Bukavu had grown into a colonial outpost in what was then known as the Belgian Congo.

Bukavu sits on the far eastern flank of this vast territory, an area the size of western Europe or the United States east of the Mississippi River. Congo is just south of the equator, close to the middle of the world and the heart of Africa, though it never feels this way. Few places have been as fascinating, and become the subject of such dark fantasies, as Congo yet been so misunderstood and overlooked.

As she faced the lottery of childbirth, what went through my mother's mind as she found herself doubled over in pain or resting between contractions on one of the thin mattresses stuffed with raw cotton that we used to sleep on at the time? Did she allow herself to think of her own mother, who had died after giving birth to her twenty-three years previously? That loss, more than anything else, had shaped her hardscrabble childhood and her stubborn personality.

Her marriage, too, had been influenced by this bereavement. My father's mother had also died during childbirth, meaning both of them faced deprivations, economic and emotional, as they grew up in their village of Kaziba, an arduous day's walk through plantations and forests to the southwest of Bukavu. They both had reason to celebrate the gift of having their own children but also to apprehend the difficulties of delivering them.

There are no reliable figures for the number of maternal deaths at this time in Congo, this being an area where the Belgian colonial authorities did not collect data. An estimate from the first national census carried out between 1955 and 1957 concluded that most women did not reach their fortieth birthday. Life expectancy was a mere thirty-eight years, and childbearing was a major killer.

Giving birth without medical care was, and still is for millions of women, a game of Russian roulette. My mother survived this round for me—and a further seven for the births of my younger sisters and brothers. But I nearly did not.

Several days after my birth my cries became piercingly high, then feeble. My skin turned pallid and my body grew feverish. When I refused to feed, it was clear I was gravely ill. My mother, still recovering from the delivery, knew she needed to act quickly and would have to do so alone. Papa was reachable only by letter.

She bundled me up in one of her *pagnes,* the colorful patterned fabric wraps worn as dresses in Congo, and strapped me to her back, my limp and burning torso pressed tight against her. She left my two sisters, then ages three and seven, with the neighbors again and headed off down the hill outside our home. Her destination was one of the only two medical dispensaries accessible to the Black population in Bukavu at the time, and she knew that being admitted would be difficult.

Both were run by Catholics, and relations between them and Protestant families like ours were still tense. The Catholic Church was one of the pillars of the Belgian colonial system, along with the state administration and the private concessionary companies that were given free rein to organize, police, and extract from large swaths of the country.

Competition between Catholics and Protestants stretched back to the first wave of European arrivals in the late 1870s and 1880s, at the start of the "Scramble for Africa," the competition among colonial powers for territory and resources. Young white traders and soldiers set out for adventure, lured by accounts of bountiful ivory and abundant precious stones, while in London, Paris, Berlin, Lisbon, and Brussels politicians schemed, plotted, and waged war to thwart their rivals.

A separate and just as consequential scramble also began: one for African souls. In the footsteps of the colonial merchants, vigilantes, and slave traffickers followed the first priests and pastors: evangelicals concerned not with the pursuit of material wealth but with spiritual conquest—although some found themselves distracted by Congo's riches, too. British Protestants in the form of the Livingstone Inland Mission arrived in 1878, followed by Baptists and Methodists from Sweden and the United States in the years after. Two French Roman Catholic missions, including the White Fathers, were active from 1880.[1]

The space was vast, the Congolese population mostly hostile, and the dangers obvious to any proselytizer daring to set out in this huge unmapped interior. Initially there was no need for competition among the various religious orders, which all felt they were engaged in the same "civilizing" mission. But this changed in the mid-1880s.

World powers recognized the territory, initially named the Congo Free State, as under the rule of King Leopold II of Belgium. Desperate to demonstrate control over his new colony—for in reality he had established merely a handful of trading points along the Congo River—Leopold enlisted the help of Pope Leo XIII in 1886.

The pope announced that Congo would henceforth be evangelized by Belgian Catholics. The Catholic faith became a tool of the colonization process, and Protestants found themselves squeezed to the margins. This schism split the early white colonizers and Congolese society as more and more people converted to the new faith.

Racked by anxiety, carrying a sick child on her back, and desperate for help, my mother stepped into this sectarian maelstrom when she approached the dispensary, a simple two-story building that offered basic health services such as vaccinations, bandages, and antibiotics. The latter would be needed to save my life.

It was run by Belgian nuns, and my mother asked them for help. She unwrapped me, sobbing as she did so. By then I was having difficulty breathing. She urged the nuns to touch my clammy skin and inspect my yellowing eyes.

But the sisters turned her away, unmoved. The dispensary was for Catholics only, they informed her. Christianity had a history of roughly seventy-five years in Congo at the time, yet the divide had hardened into a wall so thick and insurmountable that it could decide life or death. My mother pleaded with the nurses to no avail.

Did my father's reputation play a role? Although he was out of town at the time, he had a growing reputation in Bukavu as the first Congolese Protestant pastor. My mother never knew if this explained the hostility of the nuns.

But as she trudged back up the hill in her sandals and her *pagne,* convinced I would be dead by the morning, she cried hot tears of sorrow and bitterness, and she cursed the stupidity of religious bigotry and her own powerlessness to overcome it.

As she rocked me later that evening at home, my slack body in her arms, she said she felt my life slipping away, that she was losing me under her gaze. She thought about the neighbor who had cut my umbilical cord. My mother was sure that she was responsible for the infection that had drained my body.

"I could see that she was making a mistake," she later told me. "But I was lying down, I'd just delivered you. I couldn't do anything."

From everything she has described of the symptoms and treatment, I'm almost certain that I was suffering from septicemia, a blood infection that is fatal for babies if untreated.

The most common cause of infection is the severance of the umbilical cord, either in the wrong way or with a dirty blade. Once a baby has been delivered, the correct procedure is to clamp the cord in two places to stop the blood flow in both directions, then cut it in the middle, leaving a stump of several centimeters on the baby's side.

The neighbor had sliced too close to my body, not leaving enough tissue to properly tie off the cord, which had exposed me to bacteria of all kinds. My navel had started oozing and suppurating days after my birth.

It might have been the end of me. I might have become a brief and painful memory for our family. But it wasn't my time. A second brave woman would enter my life in the first few days of my existence, prefiguring the many others I have encountered since. I owe my survival to her.

Life in Congo often depends on chance encounters. In a moment of need, you might meet a compassionate stranger; when you least expect it, a man with a gun. In a world of chronic unpredictability, the divine hand of Providence appears at work constantly, perhaps explaining why we Congolese are so superstitious and such faithful believers. We all muddle through, trying to protect ourselves and our families, our lives seeming to depend on forces beyond our immediate sight. This was as true in 1955 as it is today.

As my mother feared the knock of Death at our home, someone in the neighborhood had set in motion events that would save me. This person—we never found out who was responsible—walked to the home of a missionary and teacher who lived in a small brick house down the hill. At around three A.M., they delivered a handwritten note explaining my mother's predicament.

The missionary was from Sweden, a woman then in her late twenties or early thirties named Majken Bergman. She had elected to live in our area of Bukavu, a rare European to choose a Black neighborhood rather than the comfort and familiarity of the white center of town. In the strictly segregated society of the time, she was perhaps the only person locally who could cut through the prejudices at the dispensary.

Majken read how the newborn son of Pastor Mukwege was gravely ill and had been refused treatment. She rose immediately, dressed, and came to the house by flashlight. My mother was dozing with me in her arms. She was initially startled but then sat with Majken and recounted her despair about her experiences earlier in the day when she'd tried in vain to see a nurse.

Majken promised to help.

At first light, she headed to the other dispensary in town, where she informed the nuns that my condition was critical and argued that my death, should they refuse to admit me, would be partly their responsibility. They issued her a red emergency admission slip, which Majken carried to my mother with instructions that she should use it immediately. This document enabled her to skip the long queue outside and head with me straight to the ward.

I was immediately administered a first dose of penicillin, and the nuns asked my mother to return in another six hours' time.

During the wait to go back, my mother watched over me at home, looking for signs of improvement as my small chest rose and fell in a succession of shallow breaths. I've seen these symptoms and the anguished look of mothers searching for the dawn of recovery thousands of times since.

At the time of the second dose of antibiotics, my condition had still not improved. The nuns tried to reassure my mother. "It will change, he'll start reacting," they told her.

It was only at the end of the day, at the time of the third jab, that I started to breathe more deeply, that the mask of pain began to drop from my features. By the following morning, the fever had receded.

My mother never forgot Majken Bergman. "It's thanks to her that you're alive," she used to tell me. In 2009, when I was invited to Stockholm to receive a Swedish human rights award, my mother suggested that we invite Majken to the ceremony and the gala dinner.

She was by then a frail and elderly lady, well into her eighties, but her memories of Congo were still vivid. When we met, it was like a reunion with a long-lost grandmother. We hugged and laughed. She had become a firm friend of the family after my birth and was touched by the invitation to the ceremony. She reminded me of the games she'd played with me as a child.

My mother made a speech during the dinner and told everyone that the real star in the assembled crowd was Majken, a woman who had devoted her life to helping others and without whom none of us would have been there. Majken looked mildly embarrassed, then teary as the room thundered with applause.

My mother, who was devout to the end of her days in 2019 at the age of eighty-seven, was also convinced that my troubled birth set the course for the rest of my existence. "When we walked into the dispensary, God placed a message in your heart," she'd say. "You should help others, just as you have been helped yourself."

I've always been uneasy with the idea of fate, because I believe so strongly in the notion of human agency. God created us, I believe, but then left us free to make our own decisions. The idea of destiny implies we are somehow passive creatures, treading selected courses.

I believe we constantly face choices, to be active or passive, to follow our conscience or to ignore it, and we use this liberty for good or ill. But my mother was convinced my path was predetermined.

Perhaps she's right that the tumult of my birth and my family history had an impact on my later life. My first professional focus would be on fighting the deadly lottery of childbirth, in which hundreds of thousands of women perish around the world each year delivering new lives in unsafe conditions. Babies continue to die because of ignorance and neglect. Maternal, neonatal, and child mortality have been reduced to insignificant levels in the West, yet they continue to haunt large swaths of the planet, including Congo.

I still marvel at the courage my mother showed as she delivered me and my other siblings at home, knowing that an infection, a breech birth, or a postpartum hemorrhage could condemn her, like my two grandmothers, to death.

And I continue to admire the selflessness of Majken, who might have ignored the knock at the door in the dead of night or concluded that the life of a poor Black child who had been refused treatment once could not be saved. But she ignored the siren call of apathy or defeatism. She understood that her identity gave her power and responsibility.

My hometown, Bukavu, was originally built on five small peninsulas of land that extend like outstretched fingers into our lake, Lake Kivu. At times of strong sunshine, its waters turn a turquoise blue of the sort seen in the Caribbean or Mediterranean. In perfect stillness at the end of the day, they are a gently shifting mirror, offering up a reflection of the surrounding hills and mountains. At dusk, in a spectacle I could never tire of, they seem to glow orange, then pink, as the sun falls. Then inky blue, then ash and black and every shade in between.

It holds a magnetic and mysterious beauty. In its watery depths, there are believed to be vast reserves of absorbed methane gas, making life there almost nonexistent.

The temperature here averages a warm sixty-eight degrees Fahrenheit (twenty degrees Celsius) all year round, owing to the altitude of nearly five thousand feet (fifteen hundred meters). We have none of the stifling heat or thick humidity found in our capital, Kinshasa, twelve hundred miles to the west on the other side of the country.

We live in a permanent springtime, rarely too hot, never properly cold. Plants flower in every month. The only major variable is the rain, which starts abruptly in the wet season, sometimes with a clap of thunder. It gushes down in great sheets, then vanishes just as dramatically as it arrived. Within hours, once the clouds roll on and the strong equatorial sun returns, limp wet grass will be spiky and dry again; roads of thick mud will again be baked hard, covered in fine red dust that gathers on the hair and eyelashes.

The ruddy brown of the mud, like dried blood or deep rust, is one of the elemental colors of the limited palette of eastern Congo. It is everywhere that humankind or nature has exposed the soil. And it contrasts with the luminous green of the thick, creeping vegetation that blankets our hillsides and valleys.

I say "limited palette" because green and brown, the colors of growth and nature, so dominate in Congo. We share our home with the world's second-biggest tropical rain forest after the Amazon, an often impenetrable blanket stretching from the eastern border to the far west.

Amid the forest are dots of flowers: the yellow inflorescence of the mango tree, the purple corona of the passion fruit vine, the string of red and yellow triangles of the heliconia palm. Yet the eye is dominated by those saturated base colors, the vivid green and rusty brown.

Beneath the canopy fan out the murky streams and waterways that churn toward the mighty, curved spine of our nation, the Congo River. It begins in the southeast, makes it way northward, then bends westward in a giant arc, turning more than ninety degrees toward the Atlantic Ocean, where it empties its frothy, sediment-rich contents with such force that a vast canyon has formed in the seabed.

The landscape around Bukavu rears up abruptly from the jagged shoreline of the lake. Even the five peninsulas of the town are steep sided, a mass of ripples and ravines. Behind them, farther inland, the rock rises in ever greater folds and hills. In the far background lie the mountains—Biéga and Kahuzi at around three thousand meters high—that shift in and out of view as clouds gather around their peaks.

There are active volcanoes, too, including Mount Nyiragongo, sixty miles from Bukavu, a rumbling cauldron that erupts periodically, spewing lava and ash into the lake. It is believed that volcanic activity around twenty thousand years ago reversed the direction in which Lake Kivu drains, sending its waters southward toward Lake Tanganyika instead of north.

The landscape of my homeland and the riches that lie beneath it were shaped by tectonic activity that has invested the region with both its unique beauty and its abundant raw materials. The tearing and renewal of the earth's surface over hundreds of millions of years explains why Congo is endowed with so much mineral wealth, so tantalizingly close to the surface. One colonial surveyor called Congo a "geological scandal."

Bukavu at the time of my birth was strictly segregated in an apartheid-like system. The central European neighborhood was a place of waterfront villas, white men in suits with slicked-back hair, and women in cotton dresses. There was a soccer field, a library, and art deco buildings.

The center was built in a replica of Belgian towns—quiet, ordered, clean—only with bigger homes and tropical gardens. Grand schools set in large, leafy grounds served the children of European settlers. Our cathedral with its large, curved white arches and domed roof was added at the end of the 1940s.

Around this central area was the so-called Asian quarter, home to Indian and Pakistani merchants who lived and traded from their homes. Farther from the lake, up in the hills, were two distant Black suburbs: Kadutu, where we lived, and Bagira.

Each morning from first light, thousands of men would stream from these zones to their jobs as porters, guards, cleaners, and gardeners in the center of town or as laborers in the local brewery, pharmaceutical plant, or fabric factory. Farther out of town lay the vast commercial plantations growing citrus fruits, bananas, coffee, and tea for export.

The colonialists—*les colons,* as they are known in French—had swapped a life under leaden skies in northern Europe for the warmth of the tropics. Despite the threat of disease—malaria was still a major killer, as was yellow fever—many Europeans thought they had found paradise.

From the 1950s, adventurous foreign tourists began heading out to Bukavu for holidays, sitting under bougainvilleas and sipping imported wine in scenery that resembled a tropical Côte d'Azur. The town was known at the time, and until 1954, as Costermansville, after a Belgian officer and vice governor.

The vacationers were driven around in imported American and European cars with gleaming chrome that sped on smooth roads fringed by flower beds and palm and coral trees. Their Belgian hosts took them out on the water in their speedboats or yachts. Waterskiing on Lake Kivu was a popular pursuit.

It was cheap, safe, sunny, and exotic. When visitors tired of the lake views in Bukavu and refreshing morning swims, they could take a paddleboat to Goma at the northern tip of the lake to gaze at Mount Nyiragongo, which looms beautifully and ominously over the population. There were safaris to see gorillas, lions, and wild elephants in Virunga National Park, which contains some of the most magnificent scenery in all of Africa.

After my sickly beginnings in 1955, my early years were spent with my doting and resourceful mother, my hardworking father, and our ever-growing family. As my father's church grew, so did our social standing, which brought improved living conditions.

We moved several times and in my late childhood settled into a larger wood-clad home with electricity and running water that had been built as part of a major public works scheme by the Belgian authorities to improve the living conditions of the Black population.

I remember the wooden dining table and chairs with their cotton cushions, our sofa, and the shelves with my father's Bibles and religious books. My parents had a gramophone and radio that we would tune to the national or local Bukavu station with the aid of a large central dial. There were three bedrooms, one for my parents, one for us boys, and another for my sisters. It was rudimentary, austere, singularly lacking in the comforts of modern-day homes. But for the time, and above all for a family of our background, it was the height of luxury.

Bukavu is unrecognizable today from the town of my childhood. I still remember walking on well-maintained pavements by the side of the asphalt roads, which were so smooth I could roller-skate down them with my sister—which we did at great risk to our lives. Each home had a fruit tree planted in its garden.

Independence upended this life and the strict racial order of the era. I was five at the time and remember only fragments. I have faint recollections of being taken by my parents in 1960 to a political speech in Bukavu, the first of my life. Though the words meant nothing to me, the experience of being among a vast crowd of Congolese left a mark. The orator was the hero of the time and now an icon in parts of Africa: Patrice Lumumba, a wiry man with a goatee beard and half-framed black glasses.

Shortly afterward, sooner than anyone expected, he became the first prime minister and democratically elected leader of the independent Republic of the Congo. Seventy-five years of Belgian rule were over.

For the first twenty years of this, Congo had been considered the private property of King Leopold II, giving him vast wealth and, for a time, prestige as a great humanitarian. Once the tyranny and rapaciousness of his regime were revealed, his African estate made him an international pariah.

On the day of independence, June 30, I can remember the dancing and music. For four days, the country celebrated. The new flag—blue with yellow stars—was hung everywhere. There were fireworks and bicycle races, music and beer. The significance was lost on me, a five-year-old, but I was happy to join in the festivities.

In fact, Lumumba and the other postindependence leaders inherited a state whose coffers had been emptied and a country of fifteen million people that could count only a few dozen university graduates. Belgium left Congo woefully unprepared for independence. And the former colony would be granted freedom only insofar as its resources and territory remained accessible and firmly in the Western orbit.

When Lumumba made overtures to the Soviet Union, seeking help with a mutiny in the armed forces, immense economic problems, and a secessionist movement in the south, his fate was sealed. He spent only three months in office. Within six months, he would be dead: abducted and assassinated, with Belgian and American connivance.

At the moment of independence, while the Black neighborhoods in Bukavu celebrated, the center of town mourned and moved. Houses emptied, removal vans arrived, and there was an unusual buzz of aircraft as families scrambled for places to fly to the safety of Europe.

This was the start of a great exodus of Europeans who reacted to the growing hostility toward them, as well as reports and rumors—some true, others exaggerated—of attacks on the white community. Their time in an African idyll would be remembered with nostalgia back home.

With their departure, the country lost the vital skills, administrative knowledge, and know-how needed to run a new and immature nation-state.

My grandparents and great-grandparents had witnessed the movement in the opposite direction: the first European arrivals in our native village of Kaziba. Populated by our community, known as the BaziBaziba, the valley of Kaziba is ringed by high, forested ridges and is wealthier than others in the area thanks to the local metal industry.

The BaziBaziba were historically skilled artisans who worked with copper and iron ore to make agricultural implements and jewelry sold throughout the Great Lakes region that comprises modern-day eastern Congo, Rwanda, Burundi, and Uganda. Our other specialty was manufacturing the tools of war, such as arrowheads and spears.

This latter skill, coupled with the fiercely independent spirit of the valley, enabled the BaziBaziba to hold off raids by Arab ivory and slave traders who pushed into eastern Congo from the early nineteenth century from the east coast of Africa. But they were no match for the guns of the European invaders.

My ancestors witnessed profound economic, political, and social shock. One decree held that all the mineral riches of the substrate belonged to the new colonial administration. Local mines were thereafter the property of Leopold II's Congo Free State, and the "indigenous population" was forbidden from owning them.

At a stroke, the local metal industry was killed off. Many artisans moved into the trading of precious metals, particularly gold, which is found in abundance in the area. Still today you will see people standing knee-deep in the streams and rivers around Kaziba panning for gold.

Any traditional chief who resisted the new colonial regime, whether the government or a private concessionary company, could be sure of retribution. Our chief was banished to the village of Kalehe one hundred miles away, where he died in jail. Others were murdered outright. In each case, the effect was profoundly destabilizing for societies built around the respect and veneration of tribal figureheads, known as *mwamis*.

As a child, I remember my parents talking about the time the chief was sent away. A measure of the impact can be heard in an expression still in use in Kaziba a hundred years later: *Mboje-Kalehe* is used when someone wants to swear something is true—on pain of being banished to Kalehe.

With the withering of the local manufacturing industry, villagers were forced to buy imported machetes, metal tools, and wheels, even though only years before they had been produced locally.

The colonial system also changed gender relations in Kaziba. The Europeans brought with them a new monetary system that gradually supplanted the barter economy in which agricultural goods and cattle had served as the main means of exchange. Under the former system, women were responsible for storing and managing the family's annual farming production under the strong matriarchal traditions of the community.

With the introduction of the Congolese franc from 1887, economic power gradually switched to men. Managing money came to be seen as a male competency. And when men went to work as porters and laborers in mines or on plantations, they earned wages that they distributed and controlled. Women lost the power they had once possessed to manage the resources of the family.

The other major import was brought by a group of Protestant Norwegian evangelicals who arrived in 1921 and asked to build a mission. Their decision to settle in Kaziba would have a profound bearing on village life, and particularly on my parents and, in turn, on me.

The Norwegian delegation, with the backing of the Belgian administration, went to present themselves at the home of our *mwami,* who listened to their offer to help the village. Maybe feeling he had no choice, or motivated by a sense of hospitality, he consented to grant the missionaries a scrap of land at the far end of the valley, a swampy, uncultivated area next to the river. Knowing the difficulties they would face, perhaps our chief assumed these curious white visitors would find the privations too great and move on or return home.

With a determination he had not accounted for, and funded by their congregations back home in Norway, the missionaries gradually established a permanent presence. Viewed initially with hostility, they were able to integrate thanks largely to medicine and education.

Word soon got around that the *muzungu* (literally "white man") could heal wounds and treat fevers much more effectively than the local witch doctor with his ointments and invocations. The missionaries had antiseptics, antipyretics to treat fever, medicine for ringworm and intestinal parasites, and a stock of clean bandages.

With each visit to their makeshift clinic, they evangelized. They took a particular interest in local children, including the orphaned and those trapped in poverty such as my parents. They also built a small chapel out of wood and thereafter began a school, which for the first time offered pupils the chance to learn to read and write in order to study the Bible. Though many parents were suspicious— sending their children to school meant they were not available to work in the fields or tend to cattle—some could see the benefits of literacy.

The number of baptisms was initially low, but the congregation grew until almost everyone had converted. The missionaries, like King Leopold II and the Belgian state, saw themselves as part of a great civilizing force by which European thinking and traditions would replace backward African practices.

Before their baptism, converts were required to remove the copper and gold bracelets and necklaces passed down from generation to generation as family heirlooms. These had been part of local tradition for centuries. Converts promised to jettison their beliefs in the spirits of their ancestors and the god they had worshipped: Namuzinda, "He who is at the end of everything." The smoking of locally grown tobacco in pipes, a popular pastime for men, was seen as sinful, as was drinking banana wine.

Village life had also revolved around the Aha-Ngombe, a public place where men would meet to discuss the affairs of the village, settle disputes, and transmit the history of the area to younger generations through our oral tradition of storytelling. It was also a place of music where you could hear the local guitar, the *lulanga,* the *karhero* flute, or the *likembe,* a sort of metal handheld piano instrument. The music and our musicians were condemned as satanic.

The arrival of Christianity resulted in a rupture with this past, even though the new faith was willingly adopted by the community, including my parents. But this early form of Christianity sought not to enrich or fuse with local spiritual and social traditions but to replace and supplant them outright. It was a cultural catastrophe in many ways, in which so much of what was precious and ancient was condemned as primitive and degenerate.

I wish there could have been an accommodation, an exchange, a recognition that both sides, the European and African, could learn from each other. But that was not in the spirit of the times. Had it been, you might still hear the sound of the *lulanga* or the *karhero* in churches today, not the organ.

Papa was one of the first to convert. Born in 1922 to a poor family of former metalworkers with no cattle or land, he was orphaned at the age of four. After his mother died in childbirth, his father lived only another few years before succumbing to illness himself.

Papa was taken in by his aunt, who did her best to provide and care for him while looking after her own children. He grew up feeling like an outsider in the only home he could remember. And as he emerged as a young man, his future looked bleak: with no land, he might eke out a living as a farm laborer at best. Because he was unable to pay a proper dowry, his marriage prospects were equally dim.

The church provided the outlet. He studied at the mission school and, once baptized, stayed on with the missionaries. He became one of the first Congolese evangelists to emerge from this tiny station at the marshy end of the valley. In the early 1940s, my mother arrived as a pupil at the school at the age of ten.

She had been sent by her brothers to get an education as the youngest and weakest of the four siblings. They had all had to fend for themselves after their mother—my grandmother—died while giving birth to my mother. Their father had remarried, and his second wife had issued an ultimatum: it was either her or his previous children. She wanted nothing to do with them.

As a result, my mother was brought up by her older brothers. They would do their best to provide scraps of food, including the occasional fish or frog. She suffered from constant health problems as a child, something that would continue for the rest of her life.

At the end of her schooling, in her middle teens, she agreed to marry my father, who had by then decided to become a pastor. He continued his evangelizing in the village, but after several years he began traveling more widely, including over the border into what is now modern-day Rwanda. In the first few years of their marriage, he was away for long periods, working for a time at a Swedish-run mission on the Rwanda-Congo border. But he finally settled in Bukavu in 1949, and my mother joined him the same year.

He was the first Congolese pastor in Bukavu, and he worked initially from the homes of fellow Protestants, using the property of a local judge for a time to conduct services. As more and more people converted, they began worshipping together in public outside, in the shade of a tree in one of the Black suburbs. In the early 1950s, he and a Swedish missionary received a green light from the colonial administration to build a church.

Times were tough, both materially and spiritually. He was paid only a modest salary, and he struggled throughout my childhood to pay the school fees for all of us children. He was also caught up in the chaos that enveloped Congo in its first years of independence after 1960.

In 1961, as boy of six, I sat in his church with my mother and sisters as heavily armed troops interrupted the service and dragged out a Swedish colleague of my father's on the orders of the local governor, who wanted to accelerate the departure of European settlers.

I still recall the sound of military boots on the concrete floor, the frightened grimace of the Swedish pastor, and being too scared to turn around to look at the troops as they left. It was my first experience of violence. Papa was arrested a few days later and had a gun held to his head in the police station.

Three years later, in 1964, antigovernment rebels overran Bukavu, shooting several people in the courtyard of the church. Three years after that, it was the turn of white mercenaries to occupy the town, forcing us once again to seek safety on foot in the countryside.

Abandoning our home was a wrenching experience on both occasions, for my parents but particularly for us children. I remember the anxiety first for our safety and then about what would happen in our absence and whether we would ever go back. In 1967, our house was mistakenly bombed by a Congolese air force plane, killing two young friends of our family, Leah and Job, thirteen and twenty, who were sleeping in my room.

These events would prepare me for other evacuations and periods of exile, for there have been many since then. I lost the illusion early that my parents, or our community, and still less the Congolese state, could shield me from danger. If there is anything positive to say, it is only that it focused my mind on what was important: the health and safety of my loved ones. Perhaps this explains why I've never been interested in accumulating possessions, knowing that they could be lost at any moment.

In times of peace, Papa found himself on the front lines of the spiritual struggle that nearly cost me my life as a newborn baby. He was viewed as a threat by some Catholics, and I can still recall my terror as a child when rocks thrown from outside would land on the tin roof of the church in the middle of a service, making a thunderous crash. Sometimes the doors would be flung open and stones would be pelted at the congregation, forcing us to dive under the rough wooden pews for protection. Thefts, too, were a constant problem.

My primary schooling in Bukavu began at an institution run by Swedish missionaries, which required a uniform in blue and yellow, the colors of the Swedish flag. This made us instantly recognizable as Protestants—and a target for local Catholic boys. Returning home was like running the gauntlet—there were insults, threats, and sometimes worse—and going out to run errands was an act of courage. Nowadays this sort of daily antagonism is a thing of the past, although prejudice can still rear its head. I had to battle deep reservations among my own community when one of my daughters chose to marry a Catholic.

My father was not a fire-and-brimstone preacher of the sort found in some modern churches and on television stations. He was soft-spoken, serious, and profoundly spiritual. His authority flowed from his knowledge of scripture and the example he set with his compassion for others. He was comfortable addressing people in public and advising them in private but was also an attentive listener.

As a young boy, I would accompany him during parish visits as often as possible, particularly on Sundays. As well as officiating at his fledgling church, he was permitted to attend to a handful of Protestant soldiers at a chapel on the main military base in Bukavu. He would start at four thirty A.M. and was under strict instructions to be finished by six A.M. when the Catholic mass would begin.

We would both get up at around three A.M. in the dark and start the five-mile walk to the other end of town. After the military, we'd travel to a police compound for another service. I was constantly in my father's shadow, looking up and listening to his sermons from the front pew or carrying his brown leather bag when we were on the move.

He was always impeccably dressed in a dark suit and tie, while I was always in a short-sleeved shirt and shorts, with polished leather shoes. I'd hold his hand as we walked. Sometimes he'd give me his Bible to carry, and I'd tuck it tightly under my arm.

One of these busy Sundays changed the course of my life.

After the services in the morning, Papa went on rounds in Bukavu and would frequently stop by to visit the infirm or unwell. I always listened to him intently. He had a way of encouraging the sick to have faith, not just in God but in themselves and their ability to recover.

He would sit close and lead them in prayer. He would hold their hands or put his on top of their head, speaking softly but firmly. He would implore them to find their inner courage and ask for God's help.

He was completely committed. He'd often return late and exhausted. No caller at our home was turned away and no request for help was ever denied. He was always available, dressing and leaving at three or four in the morning if necessary to support a sick family or deliver the last rites.

And yet at some point I realized, as all boys must do about their fathers, that he had human limitations. Against typhoid, malaria, yellow fever, polio, or cholera, a whole range of pathologies that sickened people then as they do now, the power of prayer had its limits.

One Sunday evening when I was eight years old, we were called to a small family house in a poor area near our home. We were led to a brick-and-wood construction with a single living space. It was dark and difficult to see inside. In the gloom, we found a mother cradling a baby. Her child was seriously ill, which was clear even to my young eyes.

I remember the whimpers, the tense atmosphere of worry and grief. I remember being filled with intense pity for this helpless bundle and being moved by the distressing noise. The scene was reminiscent of my own sickly start in life. I wanted desperately for my father to intervene; I willed him to take away the suffering.

He listened to the family and examined the child. He offered advice in his usual fashion: the medical dispensary was closed, he said, but he suggested they go in the morning and ask for a nurse. He prayed with the family and offered reassurances. And then we left.

We took the same route back home. I was lost in my thoughts, filled with remorse for the baby as well as incomprehension and disappointment at what I had witnessed.

"Papa, why didn't you give that child some medicine like you give to me when I'm sick?" I asked after a few minutes. My words broke the silence that had settled between us since leaving the family.

My father stopped walking and turned to face me. I looked up at him, seeing his features in the light of a nearby streetlamp. Our shadows stretched out in the otherwise quiet street.

"I do what I know to do: I pray," he replied. "The people who give out medicine, the *mugangas,* have been trained to do that. That's their job."

I had no idea how doctors or nurses worked or what prescriptions were. I had only vague notions about "jobs." But I'd seen the nuns in white blouses at the dispensaries who gave the medicine to my parents when I or my siblings had fevers. In the years after my birth, they became more welcoming for people of all faiths. We called the nuns *mugangas* in Swahili, the most commonly spoken language in eastern Congo. It means "people who look after the sick."

"In that case, I'm going to be a *muganga*," I told my father a touch indignantly.

"Perfect," he replied, smiling. "We can work as a team. You'll give out the medicine and I'll pray for the patients."

It felt as though a pact had been made at that spot on the road. When we arrived home, I burst in and told my mother. I don't remember her reaction. Perhaps she smiled to herself, sensing me taking the first step toward fulfilling my destiny. She told me much later that she used to pray I would become a doctor. From this point on, I had an objective in life; whenever I faltered, my mother would remind me of it.

2

A WOMEN'S HEALTH CRISIS

*I*t would take me nearly twenty years to honor my pact with Papa. As an adult, I never did the rounds of his parish with him to visit the sick and infirm, as I had once imagined. But at the end of his career, by which time he had helped build the biggest Protestant church in Bukavu with capacity for seven thousand people, I was finally working as a doctor. In our separate ways, we were each focused on the well-being of our communities, as we had agreed, although never as the twosome of my childhood fantasies.

My first experiences came as a student doctor at a hospital run by the Swedish Pentecostal Mission in Congo, about forty miles south of Bukavu. It was in a remote village called Lemera, which is set back among hills that rise up beyond the steep-sided valley of the Ruzizi River. To reach it, I would take the bus along a slow, winding road that runs roughly parallel to the river, which forms the border between Congo and our neighbors Rwanda and Burundi. I'd stop after an hour and a half and complete the last stretch of the journey on foot—a four-hour strenuous hike up slippery paths.

The hospital comprised a series of single-story buildings, the former dormitories of a colonial-era school, built among palm trees and rich vegetation on a gently sloping plot. Staff buzzed between the separate outhouses, offering maternal health care, pediatrics, general medicine, and surgery. It had two hundred beds and was the only facility for a poor and inhospitable area of 120,000 people.

My first weeks there in 1983 were a revelation, for good and bad reasons. The hospital was chronically understaffed. There was only one overwhelmed full-time doctor, Svein Haugstvedt from Sweden, a pediatric surgeon, who was assisted by a small team of nurses. There was no soft start in a place of such few resources.

I was quickly thrown into the action. Within days, I was helping Svein and the surgical team operate on patients suffering from hernias, burns, or broken bones. Adults and children, men and women. The action was relentless.

My route into medicine had been long and tricky. Although I was prepared for the hard work, it would require more patience than I had imagined. Part of the problem was the need to negotiate the dysfunctions of the Congolese state under the dictatorship of Joseph Mobutu, a onetime journalist who had seized power during my childhood.

Despite a chronic shortage of doctors, I was unable to find a place at a medical university, and several applications for grants to study abroad were rejected, to my huge disappointment. The only course I was accepted for, in engineering at the main university in the capital, I abandoned during my second year.

I spent several years drifting in my late teens and early twenties. I started to worry that my medical ambitions were an impossible fantasy. Had my mother not intervened, I might well have become a businessman. While in Kinshasa as an engineering student, I found I had a knack for making money, first with a cart business and then trading in paper, schoolbags, and other student materials.

But my mother pushed me constantly. She reminded me of my childhood ambitions every time we spoke by phone. She used to write me letters regularly saying she feared for my future.

Her health was always frail, and at one point she called to ask me to return to Bukavu urgently, explaining that she was sick and in danger of passing without seeing me one last time. I rushed home from Kinshasa, wanting to be at her side and expecting the worst.

But by the time I arrived, she had recovered. She was back on her feet and we hardly discussed her illness. Instead, she wanted to talk to me about my career. She had found out about a new medical school that was being built in Bujumbura, the capital of Burundi, which was a half day's journey by road to the south. She used all her powers of persuasion to make me apply. She wanted me close to her, she said.

I objected on various grounds. It was a brand-new faculty of unknown quality. Having already had one false start as a student during my engineering studies, I was reluctant to risk another. I argued that I should wait and continue applying elsewhere, including in France.

But seeing her resolve, I dropped my resistance and followed her advice, telling myself that I would do a year just to give it a try.

I was accepted to the course, thanks to her, and I never looked back. Despite my initial misgivings, the quality of the teaching was exceptional.

After six years, I landed in Lemera. I arrived intending it to be a short work experience before pursuing my studies and a specialization. True to my pact with my father, I planned to become a pediatrician to be able to help young children. I had completed my medical thesis on the transmission of hepatitis from mother to child during pregnancy and the vaccination of infants against hepatitis B.

But the time I spent in Lemera left an indelible mark. I saw with my own eyes for the first time the extent of the maternal health-care crisis in rural Congo.

There was almost no prenatal care, and the vast majority of mothers in the area gave birth at home, with no medical expertise at hand, just as my mother had for me in 1955. The scale of the losses and the courage of the extraordinary women I encountered made me reconsider whether I wanted to become a pediatrician.

I sensed, too, that the lack of maternal health care was symptomatic of something larger: that the lives of women were taken for granted and seemed to be undervalued. Everyone around Lemera, and most of the population of Congo, faced a battle with extreme poverty. But the hardships were not equally distributed.

Women grow up in Congo being treated as second-class citizens from birth, as they are in most societies to varying degrees. In rural areas, as well as delivering and caring for children, they are expected to do most of the work in the fields, producing staple crops such as the cassava we use to make flour or the charcoal needed for cooking.

For reasons of tradition, carrying loads is also seen as a woman's domain. I had grown up seeing stick-thin women staggering with enormous canvas bags full of crops or firewood on their backs. The load, often bigger and wider than their bodies, is carried with the aid of a strap that loops from the bag and around the forehead of the carrier. The women stoop forward to support the weight, developing phenomenally strong neck muscles but also a host of musculoskeletal disorders and sometimes reproductive problems as a result.

On top of the daily grind of work and self-sacrifice, society takes no pity on them. If divorced or widowed, they have little prospect of remarrying. They have almost no economic independence and are often physically abused by their husbands, the results of which we would see at the hospital in Lemera. Some also live in fear of their husbands taking another wife and forcing them to live in a polygamous relationship, the disastrous effects of which I have heard about over my many years of listening to Congolese women.

In Lemera, I saw the consequences of the neglect of women at the moment of childbirth, when they are at their most vulnerable and most powerful—when our Creator, through the design flaws of human anatomy, forces them to risk their own lives to deliver new ones.

Families would arrive carrying barely conscious pregnant women slung on makeshift stretchers fashioned with tree branches and string. Other times patients would simply be deposited on clotted and blood-soaked blankets outside the hospital. Their agonizing journeys had usually taken hours, sometimes days.

Many of the women had suffered obstructed labor at home, with the fetus stuck in the pelvis or partially exposed from their vulvae;

others were hemorrhaging, the biggest postpartum killer world-wide and a particular danger for very young mothers.

It was often too late to do anything other than record the cause of death. Many patients had breathed their last as they were being jolted along jungle paths and over streams on the way to the hospital. Some would arrive alive but with their uterus in a state of putrefaction days after a failed delivery. Swarms of flies would sometimes follow me into the operating theater.

I was shocked by the level of damage. Death lingered over our work at all times. We scrambled to keep it at bay. On many days I'd perform three and sometimes four emergency cesarean sections. I quickly became adept at treating women in shock caused by blood loss. Our stock of oxytocin, a drug used to stimulate contractions of the uterine wall to close the arteries during a postpartum hemorrhage, saved lives every day.

I also discovered for the first time the personal devastation caused by an obstetric fistula. These commonly occur during obstructed labor when the pressure of the baby's head restricts the blood flow in the tissue separating the vagina and rectum, or the vagina and bladder, or sometimes both. The lack of oxygen causes necrosis in the tissue, which eventually disintegrates, opening up a hole between these cavities.

As a result of the damage, women find themselves unable to control their urine and feces. The contents of the bladder or rectum leak into the vagina. It is humiliating and makes it impossible for sufferers to keep clean. The smell often leads to them being divorced and ostracized by their communities.

The tissue does not grow back on its own and can be repaired only with complex gynecological surgery. Although obstetric fistulas have been virtually eliminated in the rich world thanks to prenatal care and cesareans, the World Health Organization (WHO) estimates that more than two million young women live with the condition in Asia and sub-Saharan Africa.

In Lemera, I felt like a rookie thrown into a dizzying and complex organization that ran on adrenaline. My actions could be, and often were, the difference between life and death. I was expected to catch up fast and take on responsibility. In fact, the speed of my promotion was a little too quick for my liking.

After around three months of work, I was at Svein's house one evening having dinner with him and his wife. He told me that he needed to leave the coming weekend to visit his children because of an unspecified problem.

"I need someone to take responsibility while I'm away. Would you be okay to be acting medical director until I come back?" he asked.

"The whole hospital?" I asked.

"Yes," he said, nodding.

"How many days?"

"I'll leave Friday evening and be back on Monday," he replied.

I didn't feel I had a choice. I was flattered, of course, but also extremely nervous.

On the Friday night after my final round of the wards, I walked to my accommodation, a small detached house next to the hospital. Dinner was waiting for me on the table, prepared by the hospital cook: rice, fried plantain, vegetables. Sometimes there'd be some goat meat. The dishes were cold, as they always were by the time I got home. I picked at them.

Then I locked my door and sat on my bed, feeling very alone. There was no telephone at the hospital. We had only a radio transmitter— the "phonie," we called it—which we used to receive and send messages at specified times of the day. I slid into bed, my mind buzzing with worries, before physical exhaustion overwhelmed me.

The respite was short. I was shaken from sleep by a forceful knock at the front door, and I scrambled for my flashlight in the pitch black, then pulled on a crumpled shirt. I could tell it was late: it was silent outside. Even the insects were resting. I opened the door and found one of the hospital guards standing in the dark with a note in his hand.

"Emergency, sir," he said as he handed me the piece of paper. It shone brightly in the flashlight beam, making me squint as I read. A woman had been admitted by the night nurse with severe bleeding. "Ruptured uterus suspected."

I stiffened. I'd never treated that condition on my own. It's rare, but one of the most catastrophic events in the field of obstetrics. Unlike a cesarean, which is a simple and well-codified procedure, it requires experience. Each one has to be tackled differently. If confirmed, it would require a complicated intervention.

I threw my clothes on and changed into scrubs as soon as I reached the hospital. I ordered our electrical generator to be fired back up—it ran for only twelve hours a day and was switched off at night to conserve fuel. For minor overnight emergencies we'd often work with battery-powered lights. The guard went to wake up the anesthetist and lab assistant, who arrived within minutes.

The patient was wheeled into the surgical bloc in a state of shock. Several blood bags arrived from the laboratory. We started transfusing immediately and put the woman under general anesthesia. We needed to bring her blood pressure up as a matter of urgency and find the source of the bleeding.

I performed a midline laparotomy, a large central incision that opens up the abdomen, and began aspirating the blood. My worst fears were confirmed. How I wanted Svein to be there! It is one thing to operate with the backstop of a more experienced mentor, quite another to act alone.

Uterine ruptures, when the uterine wall tears during delivery, are caused when the fetus cannot be expelled. The baby was lost, but the mother still had a chance of survival.

I faced a choice: either attempt to repair the uterus by suturing the tear, which would give the woman a chance of having other children in the future, or perform a hysterectomy, removing the uterus entirely, which is a simpler operation with a higher chance of success.

She was visibly young, and this was perhaps her first delivery. I felt a great weight of responsibility, as if I held her destiny in my hands. I knew the impact of depriving a Congolese woman of her ability to reproduce: being a mother is unfortunately often the only way to find a place and status in society.

I opted to repair the tear and asked for my surgical books to be brought from my room. I would spend the next three hours poring over a chapter that explained the technique.

I must make a special mention here of my assistant that evening, Epike. As my gaze flitted between the patient and the pages of my manual, he monitored her blood pressure, held instruments for me, and directed the light. We are still working together nearly forty years later. He's now in his seventies but is still traveling with mobile health-care teams to remote areas of the country.

The operation was laborious and nerve-racking. Once I'd finished, I went back to bed to get a few hours' sleep, fearful of what I would discover in the morning. Had I made the right decision? Perhaps I should have just performed a hysterectomy after all?

When I woke up in the morning, she was the first patient I went to visit. I found her conscious and asked the nurse for her parameters. Her blood pressure was at a healthy level; there was some blood in her urine, but not at alarming levels; her condition seemed stable. At that moment, I felt like the happiest man in the world. With my limited experience, I had saved a life and perhaps, if she recovered fully, offered her an opportunity to have other children.

My time in Lemera was filled with such moments of drama, of snap decisions with life-altering consequences. There were constant knocks on the door at night. My days were an exercise in managing emergencies and prioritizing needs. Over the course of the year, my weight dropped to around 120 pounds, the lowest it has ever been—the result of too many missed lunches and evenings of picking at cold food before I collapsed into bed.

There were miracles, women who looked beyond salvation but who came back from the dead. I remember one in particular who went into cardiac arrest during a hysterectomy. I watched as her pulse slowed, then stopped, and the bleeding ceased completely. We gave her a fresh transfusion under high pressure and the anesthetist administered cardiopulmonary resuscitation: just as we were losing hope, her heart began beating again.

Other days were harrowing. I'll never forget a widow who ar-

rived with her barely conscious adult daughter who had hemor-
rhaged while giving birth. As we battled to save the patient, I could
hear the shrieks of the distraught mother outside.

"She's my only child. . . . Please, please, Doctor! Please save
her!" she was shouting hysterically between great sobs.

It was hard to concentrate as we tried to reanimate the patient.
At one point, the mother banged on the door of the operating theater, demanding to be let in. If her daughter had given birth in the
hospital, her life would have been saved with a simple cesarean.
But we lost her.

I had to go outside and inform the mother. It was like witnessing
another life shatter before my eyes. She left and never came back
to claim the body of her daughter. Perhaps her grief was too great,
perhaps she no longer had the strength to keep living herself.

I was filled during this period with a swirl of different emotions.
I developed profound admiration for the women in the communities
we served around Lemera, how they faced pregnancy and childbirth so stoically and in such precarious conditions. But I also felt
pity and anger that they were so abandoned by a government that
failed to provide the facilities needed to allow them to deliver in
safe conditions.

It occurred to me that the reason they were so neglected was a
reflection of their lowly status in society. Dying in childbirth was
one of the many hazards women were expected to face quietly and
without credit. The risks were ignored by men.

Almost all pregnant women who came for a consultation would
be accompanied by their mothers or mother-in-laws, never their
husbands. Those suffering complications in midlabor or in need of
emergency care would be carried to the hospital by men, often by
their spouses, but their involvement would end there. Almost none
would stay to witness the birth or the recovery.

Fathers remain absent for almost all births in Congo even today,
as they were in the Western world until a few generations ago. And
men are reluctant caregivers for their children thereafter. This pattern is repeated in almost all highly patriarchal societies.

I used to talk to my patients in Lemera about their husbands, and more recently, I've made my own modest attempt to change attitudes in my current hospital by building private rooms where women can give birth with their partners present. Sadly, I've made little progress.

The biggest objection is that it is not traditional for men to be present at the moment of birth and that they shouldn't see their wives naked and vulnerable. Others worry that their husbands might not find them attractive afterward.

It's true that childbirth isn't sexy. There are grunts and screams, blood and fecal matter. But this attitude betrays the sexist belief that a woman should be an object of desire and pleasure for her husband at all times. And have you ever met a man who doesn't want his wife or partner by his side during a moment of physical suffering?

I've always noticed the imbalance during my work: whenever a man is admitted for a problem, he's accompanied by his wife, perhaps a sister or mother, too. When he's incontinent, his wife will bring him his pot. She'll wash him and change him. He never worries about not being attractive to her in these moments.

Attitudes to childbirth by fathers are a reliable marker of how free and respected women are in any given society. In the West, by and large, men saw childbirth as the unique responsibility of their partners until relatively recently.

Attitudes began to change only in the 1950s to 1960s, when it became commonplace for women to deliver in hospitals rather than at home. From the 1970s onward, most fathers began to be present, and nowadays the overwhelming majority attend, up to 90 percent in many Western countries. Not all of them are enthusiastic for sure, but they are nevertheless in the room offering support at the crucial moment.

At the time I was working in Lemera, my country was one of the most dangerous places to give birth in the world. Sadly, the plight of Congo's mothers has not improved since. In fact, the maternal mortality rate has worsened over the length of my career.

More women die now in Congo than they did in 1990. An estimated 850 women lose their lives for every 100,000 live births in Congo, according to the United Nations International Children's Emergency Fund (UNICEF),[1] one of the highest rates in the world. In 2018, roughly 7 Congolese children out of every 1,000 born never reached their first birthday.[2]

The cause of the maternal deaths is mostly down to the failure to provide birthing facilities for routine checkups and emergency care when needed. It is not necessarily complicated or expensive. Pregnant women need good diets, as well as safe water and sanitation, but above all they need a midwife and a surgeon on hand at the critical moment.

Worldwide, one in five pregnant women continues to deliver as my mother did for me in 1955—without a skilled health professional in attendance. In sub-Saharan Africa, the numbers are even worse. Four out of ten women give birth without medical care.[3] This abandonment is a form of violence against women.

At a global level, the world has made progress, having made maternal health one of the UN Millennium Development Goals at the turn of the century. The death rate per 100,000 births has fallen by around 30 percent since the year 1990.[4]

Fortunately, there are very few countries that have as poor a record as Congo. All developed countries made even further improvements over the twenty-five-year period between 1990 and 2015, roughly halving the already low number of women who die during childbirth. Most deaths in the rich world—there are between 3 and 8 per 100,000 births depending on the country—are caused by preexisting and unrelated medical conditions.

The United States is one of the countries, like Congo, that has gone backward. The number of women dying during childbirth rose from 17 per 100,000 in 1990 to 26 per 100,000 in 2015—roughly the same level as in Uzbekistan or Kazakhstan, worse than China with its billion-plus population, and worse even than sanctions-hit Iran.[5]

The main reason is the shocking death rates for Black and Native American women. Black pregnant women are three to four times more likely to die during pregnancy than their white peers, according to data from the Centers for Disease Control and Prevention, the US public health watchdog.

Around forty Black women die per 100,000 births in the United States, a mortality rate comparable to Mexico's or Egypt's.[6] In New York City, Black mothers were twelve times more likely to die than white mothers, according to data from the city's health department.[7] Racism and prejudice play a part in explaining this gap, as does the increased likelihood of Black women lacking medical insurance and being sufferers of chronic diseases such as obesity or hypertension.

While working in Lemera, I also perceived for the first time another common form of mistreatment of mothers. It was less visible than the bruises and cuts caused by domestic battery, and less catastrophic than obstructed labor or postpartum hemorrhaging, but it was a form of violence nonetheless.

All pregnant women were expected to toil in the fields almost until their first contractions. They worked until they could no longer physically stand. There was no letup from the planting, cultivating, and carrying, on top of their domestic chores and duties. And as soon as they had delivered, the backbreaking routine resumed.

The world has made great strides here, too, in recognizing that delivering a baby is a physically exhausting and sometimes dangerous act that needs to be protected. Most societies can also see the value in a new mother being able to spend time with her newborn after giving birth, which has led to the development of parental leave.

There are only two countries in the world that do not mandate a form of paid maternity leave for workers, according to the Organisation for Economic Co-operation and Development (OECD) and the International Labor Organization.[8] The Pacific island of Papua New Guinea is one of them. The other is the United States, although President Joe Biden has announced plans to finally address this anomaly with his American Families Plan.

Only 19 percent of American workers have access to paid parental leave, and the figure is even lower for Black or Latina mothers, US Department of Labor figures show.[9] An estimated 25 percent of American mothers return to work within two weeks of giving birth, according to the advocacy group PL+US (Paid Leave for the United States). Such needless suffering for mother and child!

The average amount of paid maternity leave offered in other industrialized, democratic countries around the world is eighteen weeks. Estonia, a tiny European Union member in eastern Europe, leads the field, offering up to eighty-five weeks of leave to mothers at full pay.[10]

Most countries have now moved on to addressing the inherent sexism of their parental leave policies: that they offer more time to mothers, who are assumed to be the primary caregivers, than to fathers. Scandinavian countries are setting the example here, making their parental leave policies gender-neutral and sometimes forcing men to make use of their rights.

The advantages for society are huge. Fathers who care for children early tend to stay more involved as children grow up and enjoy improved mental health.[11] Research also shows that a father's involvement at birth and in the early years increases his willingness to share domestic tasks afterward, reducing the burden of cleaning, cooking, and washing that falls overwhelmingly on women.

As a student doctor working in a rural hospital in eastern Congo, I didn't fully understand the connection between everything I was seeing—the endless work for women, the lack of medical care, the absent fathers, the callous treatment of new mothers, the needless deaths. I didn't yet understand how our patriarchal system shaped our social norms, the economy, family life, and policy making. I was just a doctor, performing my duties, intervening where I could to help patients.

But I was aware of the injustice. The inequality troubled me. I decided that I wanted to help. Although society looked down on these women as inferior and weak, I witnessed their strength in the face of pain and uncertainty on a daily basis.

In retrospect, I see I was taking the first steps toward developing a feminist conscience. I was starting on a journey of learning and understanding that has continued my whole life.

I knew that there wasn't a single fully qualified gynecologist in the whole of our province of South Kivu at the time, let alone in the Lemera area. Women died every day for want of a simple cesarean. Suffering a fistula often meant a lifetime of stigma and rejection. The closest facility for treating them was in Addis Adaba in Ethiopia.

I considered the idea of abandoning my plans to study pediatrics in favor of gynecology and obstetrics, which for me was simply a different way of caring for children. I was married by this time, and the support of my wife, Madeleine, was essential. One of my professors warned me that working in gynecology could take a toll on relationships. He told me several male colleagues had suffered unhappy marriages as a result.

I had first briefly encountered Madeleine during a summer break back home after my first year of studying in Bujumbura. We chatted for just a few minutes outside my parents' house along with some other friends. I was struck by her smile and poise, her grace and warmth. She had an extraordinary effect on me. My heart raced, and my imagination took flight.

My excitement was equal to my disappointment afterward when I discovered that she was, as my friend Sylvan informed me, "the daughter of Kaboyi." Kaboyi was one of the wealthiest traders in Bukavu. His status placed Madeleine far beyond my reach.

I had to wait a year before meeting Madeleine again. The following summer, we were both guests of honor at the wedding of mutual friends. She was twenty; I was twenty-five. The marriage was taking place at my father's church and we were reunited there for rehearsals.

On the day itself, the groomsman who was meant to walk with Madeleine never arrived. We waited until the final minutes before the start of proceedings, at which point I was asked to take his place. I could barely conceal my delight.

I don't remember much about the wedding ceremony. It was long, well over two hours. I sat next to Madeleine and we chatted in hushed voices on our pew between the hymns and Bible readings.

The words just seemed to flow. We opened up to each other,

naturally and without affectation. She asked about my life in Bujumbura. She told me about her studies. I talked about my family, my first medical exams, and my dreams for the future. My heart was racing again.

Toward the end of the wedding, on a whim, acting entirely on impulse, I asked her if she would move with me to Bujumbura. I smiled wryly and expected her to demur. To my surprise, she accepted with a whispered "Sure, why not?" and laughed.

I fell helplessly and irredeemably in love with her at that moment. We spent another two hours talking after the ceremony outside the church and then began seeing each other over the summer. We made a pact: if anyone tried to oppose our relationship, which we anticipated, we would work to overcome them.

I informed my parents soon after about my intentions: they were skeptical but not opposed. Madeleine's family was far more difficult to convince. Her father wondered how a medical student and the son of a pastor was going to provide for his daughter, who had been brought up in the most comfortable conditions money could buy in Bukavu at the time. But Madeleine would not be discouraged. She was true to our pact, and he eventually relented.

In 1980, a year later, we were married at my father's church. My family provided the dowry—four cows. Shortly after, we moved to Bujumbura together and started a family in a modest rented home.

Everything I've achieved and endured since has been with Madeleine. We've celebrated all the triumphs, lived the fears, and felt the darkest moments of grief together; we've laughed and we've despaired; we've traveled and discovered the world, raised children, and grown older together. For forty years, we've been on the same path, side by side.

In 1984, as my time in Lemera was drawing to a close, I asked Madeleine if she would support me in studying obstetrics and gynecology, which would require her to move again. I had been offered the possibility of a place at a medical university near the wine-growing region of the Loire Valley in central France. If I passed the entrance exam, I'd be admitted on a four-year course.

Madeleine agreed. I had $2,000 in savings at the time, half of which went for the airfare to Paris.

I arrived in October on my first trip to Europe. I landed at Charles de Gaulle Airport to the northeast of the city and made my way to Montparnasse in the south, where a family friend had agreed to pick me up in his car. He drove me to the small town of Angers, which would be my new home.

I left for France on my own on the understanding that once I had established myself, Madeleine would join me along with our two young children at the time. My first task was finding an apartment, which proved more difficult than I imagined.

I scoured the local newspaper for rooms to rent. But when I'd arrive for viewing appointments, I'd be told the place had just been let. Only after numerous failed attempts—and the realization that places I had visited were still being advertised the day after—did I suspect that the color of my skin was causing such problems.

It was a frustrating and dispiriting experience, but it came to an end one day when I rang for a spare room in a shared house with two other students and introduced myself immediately as a Congolese medical student. "Fantastic. What time do you want to visit?" replied the landlord, Paul, who would become my local guide and a dear friend throughout my time in Angers.

The first two months were a difficult period. I had major financial worries, which came to an end only when I won a small French car in a raffle at a local supermarket. It allowed me to take up the offer of paid shifts at the hospital and others in the area. This incredible stroke of luck set the tone for the rest of my time in France.

It was a happy and hugely fulfilling period of our lives. Madeleine moved over and we had a third child while living in Angers. We had wonderful friends, and despite my initial encounters with bigoted landlords, we were made to feel tremendously welcome.

Some of my professors were surprised at my level of experience. I remember in particular assisting one of them during a cesarean. When you're working with an assistant, it becomes clear very quickly how confident they are and their level of proficiency. At one point, he turned toward me with a quizzical look on his face.

"Have you done this many times before?" he asked.

"About five hundred," I replied.

I wasn't being boastful: it simply reflected the demands of the work at the hospital in Lemera.

The professor looked startled.

"Then why are you here?" he asked.

"I've still got lots I want to learn," I replied.

When I told colleagues in Angers how sometimes I'd have to administer anesthetics myself back home, they couldn't believe it. None of them could fathom how we'd worked by flashlight if the generator wasn't running or how I'd once operated on a uterine rupture while consulting my manuals. I was living and working in a different world now, seeing the incredible inequality of global health care before my eyes.

In all my time in France, I never witnessed a woman die from childbirth. Not once.

The maternity wing of our hospital in Angers could count on around thirty doctors, including obstetrician-gynecologists and neonatal resuscitation specialists. There were dozens of midwives, as well as secretaries and other support staff. There was a full delivery team present twenty-four hours a day. Each patient would undergo a battery of prenatal tests, the expense of which was all covered by the public health system.

I discovered at some point that the number of babies born in the maternity unit in Angers—roughly thirty-five hundred a year—was the same as we were delivering in Lemera with just two doctors and eight midwives.

In Lemera, I'd sometimes ask my patients to undertake simple urine or blood tests, and many would reply that they couldn't afford it. In Angers, there were diagnostic machines worth hundreds of thousands of dollars that were barely used.

I remember being astonished at how surgeons in France would

take a new roll of thread for each suture. They'd often use just part of it and toss the remainder at the end. I had the habit of using every last wind of material.

At the end of my five years of training, we faced a choice. We could stay in Angers and continue to enjoy the comfortable life we had created for ourselves. I had job offers and opportunities; the children were in great schools; Madeleine had used the time to complete her own studies in tropical medicine. Or we could return to Congo, where things had grown much worse in our absence.

Mobutu, who had renamed the country the Republic of Zaire and insisted that everyone use traditional Congolese names and dress, was plundering the country. His economic policies—above all, nationalizations that had seen companies carved up and distributed to his cronies—spelled disaster. Mining output fell, cutting the main source of wealth for the nation. As government resources shrank, he printed money, creating hyperinflation and hardship.

The economic infrastructure left by the colonial administration had also fallen into permanent disrepair. Roads and railways rotted. Mobutu had no need for them, as he flew everywhere by private jet or helicopter.

As we contemplated returning, schoolteachers nationwide went on strike because they hadn't been paid. Hospitals found themselves unable to buy medication. Corruption had become endemic and was officially endorsed. "You have guns, you don't need a salary," Mobutu once told his security forces.[12]

I had to weigh my commitment to the mission I had developed for myself—returning to help the women of Congo—against the needs and desires of my family. I knew other foreign medical students at the time who decided to stay in France. Some of them remain friends. I understand and make no judgment on their choices.

But at a global level, the consequences of the medical brain drain from poor to rich countries are significant and are an important part of the picture of global health and economic inequality today.

The emigration of medics from the developing world to the developed world deprives poor countries of much-needed skills. In the United States and the United Kingdom, there is roughly one physician for every four hundred people, while the wealthiest European countries such as Germany or Sweden have one for every two hundred people, according to WHO data. In Congo, there is barely one doctor for every ten thousand citizens.

Each time a doctor trained in Africa or in another developing nation is recruited in North America or Europe, it worsens the imbalance in care and represents a cost saving for the rich host country, which often paid nothing for that doctor's training.

In the United States, around one in three physicians was born in another country, and almost 7 percent are not US citizens, a major study using census data showed in 2018.[13] In the United Kingdom, one in fifty members of the National Health Service staff is African, according to a 2018 parliamentary report, and the recent novel coronavirus crisis, as in many other countries, has highlighted the extent to which developed countries rely on foreign-born medics.

Developing countries lack both general physicians and, even more chronic, the specialized skills that command the highest wages in the West. I was reminded of this a few years ago when a Congolese oncologist contacted me from Belgium where he had settled. His mother in Bukavu had just been diagnosed with late-stage cancer. He asked me if I could help.

I did my best to arrange some care for her. Over the course of several phone calls, he told me how he owed his education to his mother, who had sacrificed herself for him, working long days selling peanuts to pay for his school fees.

There was something desperately sad that I could hear in his voice. He was in Europe amid comfort and abundance, but the woman who had helped provide this life for him was dying back home from a condition he might have detected early and treated.

Despite all the difficulties in Congo, and the attractions of our life in France, I still felt I wanted to go back. Every time I thought about staying, my conscience felt troubled. It was as if I were abandoning an ideal. I'd picture the stretchers back in Lemera or hear the voice of that desperate mother who banged on the wall of the operating theater as I attempted to save her daughter.

I talked it over with Madeleine. She needed some persuading at first, but she understood my reasoning. We came up with a compromise: We would buy return air tickets. We'd go home for six months and reassess at the end of this period. If we were unhappy, we would come back to France.

"Are you sure you've thought this through?" my supervisor at the hospital, Roger Le Lirzin, asked me. "Are you sure you're not missing the chance of a lifetime for your children?" I thanked him for his concern. I knew he had my interests at heart, but I said my mind was made up.

We flew home and I returned to the hospital in Lemera as the first trained obstetrician-gynecologist in the region. The next few years were some of the most satisfying of my life professionally, even as the country lurched from crisis to crisis at the end of Mobutu's thirty-two-year rule.

I became medical director of Lemera Hospital. We expanded, adding another hundred beds and a separate outbuilding for radiography and another for infectious diseases. My most significant contribution was setting up a training program for midwives in the region. With this, we could reach women in the most remote areas. We also built a small training college for nurses at the hospital, thanks to fundraising from my first landlord, Paul, and friends back in Angers. We were soon producing the staff we so sorely needed.

At the hospital, we built a large area—we called it Svein Hall in honor of my former boss—where women could come to stay up to two months before their delivery date, free of charge. This meant we could ensure they were eating a balanced diet and problems were identified early and averted. It spared them from work in the fields while heavily pregnant. We had around a hundred women staying with us at all times.

Maternal death rates began to fall. I could see it in the records at the hospital. We recorded fewer fatalities; we had fewer mothers arriving in a critical state. I could also see with my own eyes how basic knowledge and education, with financial backing from our donors, was starting to transform lives. The odds of dying a painful, avoidable death while giving birth in the area around Lemera were starting to fall.

I felt the decision to return was being vindicated. It wasn't easy and came at some personal cost. I was away from my family for long periods because Madeleine and the children stayed in Bukavu. I would return home for one weekend every fortnight.

In my limited spare time, when I wasn't back home, I'd sometimes go for a hike up in the hills around the hospital to clear my head. These were the only moments when I was able to truly relax. The fresh air and nature would revitalize me. I'd always try to walk to a spot where I could look out and see the horizon, with the mountaintops and valleys stretched out in front of me.

My favorite vantage points were those where I could look down on the river Ruzizi. I would watch it weave around rocky outcrops or fork into separate streams, forming small islands surrounded by rushing water. I would listen for the faint noise of the rapids as it echoed up the steep valley sides.

From up high, I could also see where the borders of Congo and those of our eastern neighbors, Rwanda and Burundi, come together. We all share the same magnificent scenery, so rich and wild. I would feel humbled by the summits around me and the force that had buckled them into jagged teeth pointing up to the sky. Humans, with their countries and borders, their rivalries and squabbles, would seem momentarily insignificant.

3

CRISIS AND RESILIENCE

"*Y*ou're needed, Doctor, right away. It's an emergency." It was 1999, and a woman had arrived on the verge of death, but in a different setting and in radically different circumstances from those in Lemera. I was back in Bukavu, in a poor, neglected suburb called Panzi, and embarking on the biggest project of my life.

With funding from the Community of Pentecostal Churches in Central Africa,[1] we were building a new hospital from scratch. We hadn't even finished the construction work when our guard, Nandola, came running to see me to announce the arrival of our first patient. "She looks badly injured," he told me.

The paint was barely dry and there were still piles of building waste lying around on the site. Boxes of medical supplies were stacked up in the corridors of the two buildings we were in the process of renovating. We didn't even have a sterilizer for the operating theater.

But word had got out. The local community was aware of what we were doing, and much sooner than we expected, a group of men had arrived outside with a homemade stretcher carrying a woman wrapped in blankets. Seeing the desperation of the bearers and hearing the faint groans of the woman beneath the sheets, Nandola had agreed to lift the plank of wood that served as the barrier blocking off our building site from the dusty road outside.

She was carried inside and lifted off the stretcher and onto a birthing table. We hadn't even had time to set up a room for consultations. As I hurried to see her, everyone sprang into action. We were just eight at the time, including administrators, all former staff from Lemera.

We began to remove the blankets to examine the patient. She was in her midthirties and was conscious, but only just. She was bleeding profusely and in excruciating pain from what appeared to be a gunshot wound around the area of her pelvis and hip.

We needed to operate immediately. Veikko, a surgeon from Lemera, led the procedure. In any circumstances, it would have been complicated. But in a half-finished building site, his coolheadedness and skill would be especially valuable.

We had to scramble just to get our equipment set up. The operating theater was filled with items we'd scavenged from various clinics and aid agencies around the region—an operating table and scialytic lights from here, radiology and anesthesia equipment from there. At one point we had to dispatch someone by car to the city center to fetch two more blood bags because we didn't have enough. We sterilized the instruments inside a pressure cooker.

We worked on the patient for most of a long and stressful day that marked the unofficial opening of Panzi Hospital. When we'd finished in the evening, our radiologist, Mungo, agreed to stay on and monitor her overnight. We went to bed exhausted, hoping to find the patient alive and well in the morning.

When I woke up and headed to the ward, to my great surprise I found she was not alone. Mungo explained how several women in labor had arrived overnight, having been told the hospital was functioning. He had been up all night assisting with the births. Mothers were happily lying in beds cradling their infants. One of them had delivered twins.

That same day we had people queuing up for consultations, pregnant women but also men and children seeking help for a whole range of ailments. It continued like this in the following weeks. The builders and decorators labored around them, applying the final touches to half-finished bathrooms, the ward, and the work spaces.

As they waited, many of the first patients sat on benches or on piles of rubble. They passed the time chatting and eating. Thanks to the discarded nuts and seeds from their snacks and meals, we soon had plants and trees growing. Today, there's an enormous avocado tree that dates back to this period. It serves as a constant reminder of our improvised beginnings more than two decades ago.

We saved the life of our first patient. She gained strength slowly, and once she had the energy and desire to talk, she told us how she had received her injuries. She had been at home when soldiers had come to the door, she explained. They had argued and one soldier had fired through the door, hitting her in the leg.

Something didn't add up. She was vague about why they had fired at her. I would learn the full story only several months later.

The hospital was a product of circumstance and necessity. Life had changed radically since my time in Lemera. The hikes to savor the views around there, the satisfaction I felt at the time at improving the health indicators for the communities we served, were memories from a calmer, bygone era. The intervening years—from 1993 to 1999—had been filled with torment and uncertainty.

My work in Lemera was ended by a conflict rooted in ethnic tensions I had first glimpsed as a child of four, in 1959. I have a hazy recollection of the streets of Bukavu being suddenly full of families with bags on their heads and possessions piled high on carts. They spoke a different language—Kinyarwanda, not the Swahili or local dialects of eastern Congo.

Above all, I remember the musty smell of thousands of horned cattle. Great herds roamed the streets, feeding off the roadside vegetation and trampling gardens. Anxious-looking men and their wives, carrying babies or leading children, walked behind them.

As I watched these scenes unfold, another frightened young boy, a country away, was caught up in the dusty columns of people and their animals. The Kagame family with their young son, Paul, were fleeing Rwanda and heading north into Uganda. Paul's life would affect mine much later.

The cause of all this tumult was violence between the two main ethnic groups in Rwanda—Hutu and Tutsi. The Hutu formed the majority of the population but had long resented their treatment by the Tutsi, who had historically been the land- and cattle-owning class and aristocracy.

The Hutu led a series of pogroms in the lead-up to Rwandan independence against the Tutsi, forcing hundreds of thousands of them to flee and settle in Burundi, Congo, and Uganda to the north. Independence in 1962 led to elections in which the Hutu gained political power for the first time. More anti-Tutsi violence in Rwanda followed in 1963 and 1973. In Burundi, which has a similar ethnic composition as Rwanda, minority Tutsi carried out massacres of the Hutu in 1972 that some historians consider to be a genocide.

Fresh Hutu-Tutsi tensions exploded again in the region in the 1990s, first in Burundi, where the country's first elected president, a Hutu, was assassinated by Tutsi army officers, and then in Rwanda in April 1994, when a further two Hutu presidents—Cyprien Ntaryamira, also from Burundi, and Rwanda's Juvénal Habyarimana—were killed when their plane was shot down. This was the spark for the Rwandan genocide.

Their assassinations created a vortex into which my life and the lives of tens of millions of people would be inexorably pulled. The worst, most destructive passions of humanity were let loose: grievances led to murder, murder to revenge, to mass killings, mass rape, and mass torture.

Over one hundred days in Rwanda, mobs of Hutu hunted down Tutsi, or anyone who looked like a Tutsi, or anyone suspected of sheltering or sympathizing with the Tutsi. Between 800,000 to one million people died, according to the International Criminal Tribunal for Rwanda, in the most notorious episode of mass killing in the latter part of the bloodstained twentieth century.

At Lemera Hospital, we had an agreement with the International Committee of the Red Cross, which sent us patients. We began receiving men, women, and children, Hutu and Tutsi, with terrible injuries. There were people who had had their throats cut. Others had had hands or feet hacked off by machetes.

I was no stranger to violence, having witnessed it repeatedly as a child, but this was the first time I had ever treated such wounds as a doctor. Life took a sudden dark turn, diverting me from my work on maternal health care. No longer would I focus on providing safe places for women to give birth; instead I would be consumed by a struggle against a far more explicit, deliberate form of violence against mothers and daughters. All the progress—the maternity clinic, our outreach programs, the training of village midwives—would be lost in the chaos.

In the popular telling of the Rwandan genocide, the "hundred days of madness" in which Hutu slaughtered Tutsi came to an end when a Tutsi rebel army known as the Rwandan Patriotic Front, led by Paul Kagame, overthrew the Hutu extremists in power and installed a multiethnic government of national unity.

This was not the end of the killing, however, but the start of a new phase. A second wave of atrocities began immediately afterward, perpetrated by the Tutsi and forces under Kagame's command against the Hutu.

They went after the people responsible for the genocide: soldiers and army officers, politicians and local officials, and members of the militia responsible for some of the worst atrocities, the *interahamwez*. But the killing was indiscriminate, and many of the criminals, known in French as *génocidaires,* fled along with an estimated 1.5 million Rwandan refugees into Congo. The leaders escaped to Europe and Kenya.

Two years after the genocide, in 1996, the new Tutsi-led Rwandan army, acting behind a front of Congolese rebels, invaded eastern Congo in pursuit of the *génocidaires* who had settled in the refugee camps around Bukavu and elsewhere. Rather than acting to disarm and separate the Hutu militias from the civilian population in the camps, which were under UN protection, the international community had let the problem fester.

The invading Rwandan forces made hunting down the *génocidaires* their public priority. But they were also intent on regime change. Mobutu, having served as a Western ally for decades, could no longer rely on foreign support after the end of the Cold War and was seen as part of the problem.

We had sensed an invasion coming in Lemera. Rebel and Rwandan forces had been spotted crossing the border into Congo at night and heading into the hills carrying weapons and electrical generators. Artillery was being occasionally fired from positions in Rwanda into Congo.

The atmosphere at the hospital grew tense. Nervous Congolese army commanders wanted to post guards at the hospital because they were worried that we were providing health care to the rebels. I refused their request and insisted that we should be a neutral place, without weapons, that cared for everyone irrespective of their ethnicity or background. I preferred to be shut down rather than have soldiers filter my patients.

And even as some of my staff left for their own safety, I resolved to stay at my post, believing that I was safe from attack in a hospital. I was wrong.

When we were attacked, it was pure chance that I wasn't there. I owe my life to a Swedish engineer, David, who lived with us at the hospital with his wife, Astrid. Or to put it another way, I am still alive thanks to David's infected foot.

Shortly before the attack, we decided to evacuate him lest the severe infection put him in need of an amputation. Despite the obvious tensions around us, we decided to take him along the road cleaved into the valley between Lemera and Bukavu.

The journey was one of the most terrifying of my life. Our hospital Toyota Land Cruiser was attacked from over the border in Rwanda as we descended into the main valley. I can still recall the rattle of machine guns above the sound of pebbles and stones pinging off the bottom of our vehicle as we drove as fast as the potholed road would permit. I expected the car to be hit at any moment.

Crouched down in the passenger seat, with bullets flying around us, I waited for the scream, the explosion, the tire blowout that would lead us to careen to almost certain death if we lost control.

On one side of the road was a rock face, on the other a sheer drop into the river.

Miraculously, we made it to Bukavu—inspecting the car only at the end and finding that a bullet had pierced the rear end and struck the luggage.

The journey saved David's leg. He was evacuated to Sweden and hospitalized. The swelling slowly went down with strong antibiotics, but his doctors were never able to identify the cause of his mysterious infection.

The same night we arrived in Bukavu, October 6, 1996, Tutsi rebels launched an assault on Lemera Hospital, killing thirty of my patients. Some of them were shot in their beds, others fled into the surrounding forests with IV drips still dangling in their arms. They were chased down and massacred. This was one of the first acts of a dirty, brutal war. In fact, the atrocities could be said to have started here.

Three of my nurses lost their lives. They barricaded themselves into their living quarters when the attack started, but the rebels smashed through the doors and executed two of them on the spot. A third was forced to drive all of the medical supplies to a nearby village in a hospital vehicle. Once this task was completed, he was killed in cold blood.

A photograph of me that hung in my office was riddled with gunfire. Bullets were fired at my white doctor's coat, which I had hung up, expecting to be back the day after I left with David. Patients records were ripped up and strewn across the complex.

Once everything of value had been looted, the hospital became a military camp, housing the rebel forces soon to be known as the Alliance of Democratic Forces for the Liberation of Congo, and Rwandan troops.

The massacre at the hospital was the prelude to a full-scale invasion of Congo by the rebels, who were fronted by Laurent-Désiré Kabila but relied entirely on regular Rwandan, Ugandan, and Burundian forces. This invasion became known as the First Congo War.

A few weeks after the attack at Lemera, Bukavu came under increasingly heavy fire. We initially intended to stay put, fearing the worst if we abandoned our home. Our contingent of badly paid Congolese soldiers was not a reassuring presence, but we still expected them to put up some sort of a fight, enabling Mobutu's government to negotiate a peace agreement with our neighbors.

None of us imagined that the armed forces would turn and run. In the end, few soldiers were prepared to lay down their lives for Mobutu, whose health was failing. At the time of the invasion, he was out of the country receiving medical treatment.

I stayed at home with Madeleine and the children. We spent our days calling friends and listening to the news for updates on the conflict and the political situation at home. Everyone wondered what we should do, contemplating whether to run or lie low.

My hand was forced when a young man who introduced himself as a military intelligence officer came to my house to say that I needed to flee. I had never met him before, but he said he had been in a meeting during which my name had come up as a possible spy and informer for the enemy. Apparently, my decision not to allow the army to post guards at the hospital in Lemera had made me a suspect.

It was absurd and irrational, but I knew lives could be lost over such follies at times of panic. I immediately bought an air ticket to fly to Kinshasa, where I knew I would be safer. We asked an influential friend of Madeleine's father, a military magistrate, to drive me to the airport in the trunk of his car.

The following morning in the half-light of dawn, he pulled up as promised. I slipped into the trunk with a small bag and a satellite phone belonging to my church organization. It was my second nerve-shredding car journey of the month, after my ordeal with David on the road from Lemera to Bukavu. I was constantly in fear of someone opening the trunk and discovering me.

It was the rainy season and a storm had drenched the city overnight. As I cowered in the back, I was able to hear the wheels skid and the splashes of puddles as we negotiated potholes and water channels. I could make out the sticky sound of the mud on the tires and wheel arches.

I bounced along in the back, my heart racing, my stomach stiff with anxiety each time we slowed down for a checkpoint.

Once we got to the airport, it was no better. It was a scene of utter chaos. There were jams of vehicles, civilian and military, and hundreds of people making their way with bags toward the single departure terminal. Crowds spilled out into the car park. Inside the terminal, there were groups of tense-looking soldiers carrying weapons.

I found a hiding place behind some containers where I could see the runway. When my plane to Kinshasa arrived, as soon as it came to a standstill in front of the terminal, passengers and soldiers rushed forward to secure seats. In the resulting stampede, people with tickets remonstrated with the troops and tried to block them. Several were shot on the spot. I saw at least three people killed like this. Groups of men in khaki fought their way up the stairs and into the plane, holding their guns above their heads.

I didn't even try to board. It became clear to me that the army was mutinying and, if so, that Bukavu would soon be defenseless. I took out my phone and dialed a colleague, Roland, another Swede working for our church organization in eastern Congo. He had flown out the week before and was in safety in Kenya.

He agreed to send a plane through the Mission Aviation Fellowship, an organization that supports church-run humanitarian groups. It sent a twelve-seater aircraft. I rang Madeleine and told her to pack bags, then called another friendly military officer and asked if he could bring my family to the airport in my car.

We all joined up behind the containers and waited for our plane. A full-scale evacuation was underway by this time. Small chartered aircraft sent by foreign governments, aid agencies, and businesses were landing regularly. My biggest fear was that as soon as our plane landed it might be swamped by desperate people or hijacked by soldiers. There was also a risk someone might get left behind in the commotion or even killed, given the shootings that I had witnessed earlier.

We scanned the cloudy sky above for what seemed like an eternity. Finally, once it had come into view, landed, and taxied to the far end of the runway as agreed, we dashed out, leading the children by the hand. It was a run of several hundred meters.

We threw ourselves inside, each person scrambling in. I counted Madeleine and the children. As soon as the seats were all full, we slammed the door shut and shouted, "Go, go, go!" The engines whirred back into life.

Once inside, I felt huge relief but also fear and deep sadness for my stricken hometown, which would be taken over by the rebels and Rwandan forces within a day. Fleeing like this was an unpleasant echo of my childhood, taking me back to the three separate times we had been forced to escape from rebels and mercenaries.

As we took off and circled northward, it was clear that a humanitarian disaster was in the making. Columns of people on foot or piled into overloaded vehicles were fleeing Bukavu, heading in the direction of the city of Kisangani four hundred miles away to the northwest.

Half a million individuals were on the move with little food or water. Many of them were Hutu Rwandan refugees from the camps around Bukavu. They feared exactions from the invading Tutsi forces, rightly as it turned out.

The Rwandan troops made no distinction between Hutu refugees and Hutu rebels in Congo. Some of those killed were extremists, no doubt, but many of the victims were innocent women, children, and the elderly who were killed ruthlessly with guns, machetes, stones, and rifle butts. Thousands of Congolese civilians running for their lives were also massacred, including more than a hundred in my native village of Kaziba. Others would die of disease and hunger as they trekked through dense jungle.

My extended family was caught up in the chaos. My father-in-law, whom I knew as an energetic man of sound constitution, was never the same after the 250-mile journey by foot he was forced to make. He and my mother-in-law drank untreated water from rivers along the way, which made them sick, and survived by foraging for fruit in the forest. Seeing them so exhausted and desperate, villagers would sometimes take pity and give them leftover rice or cassava.

With his wealth, my father-in-law was able to pay for specialized medical care afterward in Kinshasa and abroad, but he never recovered fully. He died at home a few years later at sixty-seven, having never regained his strength. My mother-in-law and brother-in-law, who had walked the same route, also died in similar circumstances.

We flew about three hundred miles north to the small Congolese town of Bunia, knowing that we were among the lucky few to have escaped. We then traveled on to the Kenyan capital of Nairobi.

The rebels and their foreign backers advanced from east to west over seven months, massacring tens of thousands of Hutu and Congolese civilians. Some Congolese wrongly saw the invading forces as liberators from Mobutu's decrepit and corrupt regime. He was overthrown in May 1997 and died four months later.

Rebel leader Kabila, an aging Communist revolutionary who had once worked with Che Guevara, was installed as president. But Rwanda, a country about one-hundredth the size of Congo, held the real power. Kabila was advised and closely watched over by Rwandan and Tutsi officers who took key roles in his administration and the armed forces.

Kenya was my home for a year, and I worked on the refugee crisis in Congo from there, attempting to draw attention to the humanitarian disaster on the ground while growing more and more distressed at the inaction of the international community. Bukavu, meanwhile, was occupied by Rwandan soldiers, and any sense of relief at the end of Mobutu's time in office proved short-lived.

Memories of the mistreatment, humiliations, and insults experienced by many Congolese during this period remain fresh. Some Rwandan soldiers used a whip as a form of public discipline, which brought back the worst memories of the colonial era when the *chicote,* a heavy lash made from the hide of the hippopotamus, was the favored means of punishment by Belgian officers.

After a year in Nairobi, I returned to Bukavu in 1998 for the first time on a fact-finding mission to check on living conditions in the city. At the end of my visit, I attempted to cross into Rwanda in order to take a flight back to Kenya. At the border, I was stopped by a guard.

"We've got orders to prevent you from leaving," he said, looking at my passport.

I attempted to reason and find out why I was being blocked. But it was futile trying to reason or argue. I trudged back to our old family home in Bukavu and called Madeleine to explain that I would not be returning that evening.

From then on, I was put under surveillance and had soldiers tailing me. At one point, I was warned by a local human rights worker, Pascal Kabungulu, that I was on a list of potential dissidents. I needed to be careful, he said. I took his advice very seriously and watched my step. Pascal was later gunned down in his home by men in military uniforms.

After several months, my family was allowed to travel from Nairobi to join me. That was the point at which I started thinking about setting up a new hospital in Bukavu.

I felt trapped. I was still struggling to process the losses in Lemera, above all the lives of the three nurses who were killed, but also my patients and the hospital itself, which was the only facility for the community.

I thought I had found a new vocation in Kenya doing humanitarian aid work around the region, including in war-torn southern Sudan. Now this life had been shut down, too. The only possibility I saw for myself was creating something from scratch.

We identified the suburb of Panzi in Bukavu as the site for a hospital because of the obvious needs of the local population and the fact that it was one of the fastest-growing areas of the city. It was a southern suburb, five miles from the center of town, along a cratered mud road that was virtually unpassable without a 4x4. In the dry season, each vehicle would kick up great clouds of dust; after rain, they slipped and splashed through huge puddles that were sometimes a foot deep.

More and more people were flooding into Bukavu at that time, making new homes for themselves after being driven from the countryside by the fighting and insecurity.

We initially planned to open a field hospital in Panzi on some land that had once been a plantation owned by colonial-era Belgians. Since then, it had been used as a military garrison but had been left abandoned before my church organization acquired it. When I first visited, there was still land under cultivation, fields of cassava and corn, as well as patches of jungle.

Every inch of available ground in Panzi has since been built on. The whole city has been transformed over my lifetime. The order and abundant wildlife and nature of my childhood are distant memories. Trees have been chopped down and burned as firewood. The flower beds and smooth roads are long gone.

The biggest changes have come in the last twenty-five years. It started with the influx of refugees after the Rwandan genocide in 1994, but the decades of war since then have led thousands of new people each year to seek security in its slums. The population has more than tripled in twenty years, leading to a wave of new construction that has washed up from the lake shoreline and all the way to the summits of the hills that overlook the city.

Our initial ambitions for the hospital were fairly modest. We would start small and then try to scale up. To begin with, we needed a birthing area and an operating theater where we could perform cesareans and other basic surgery. We planned to offer general health services, but with a focus on my area of expertise in maternal health.

Any woman who encountered difficulties during labor in the Panzi area back then needed to travel all the way across town to the public hospital, the only one for Bukavu's population at the time of five hundred thousand people. This journey, by foot or taxi, was hazardous and sometimes fatal, with delays caused by the numerous military checkpoints of that era that needed to be negotiated.

I remember visiting the public hospital around this time. I accompanied the pregnant wife of a friend of mine and was horrified by what I saw. At the entrance to the maternity wing, several women were inconsolable, having just lost a pregnant relative during childbirth. They were on the ground, beating the pavement with their hands between shrieks of pain. A second woman died during a C-section while I was there.

We negotiated with UNICEF to secure tents for our use, and we sourced operating equipment from Austria. In July 1998, we persuaded the governor of South Kivu and the mayor of Bukavu to attend a ceremony to mark the start of work to prepare the site.

It was all very low-key—we had a choir sing and a few speeches—and there was a sense of urgency. We needed our VIP attendees to sign the permits that we needed to start working before the outbreak of more fighting. The country was heading for another crisis.

Just over a year after replacing Mobutu, President Kabila found himself under pressure to restore Congolese sovereignty. The population was chafing under the occupation by Rwandan, Ugandan, and Burundian soldiers, and he faced protests about the presence and obvious influence of so many Rwandans in the government and armed forces.

In late July, just weeks after our ceremony at the hospital, Kabila made his move. In a public address, he thanked our neighbors for their services and asked them to withdraw their forces from Congo and leave.

Some troops were withdrawn, but Kabila's former partners saw his move as an unacceptable betrayal. Two weeks later, they returned for another invasion of Congo. It was led by the same man as the first, Rwandan general James Kabarebe. This time it was fronted by a different group of Congolese rebels, known as the Rally for Congolese Democracy (RCD). The fighting started in August 1998 and became known as the Second Congo War.

The public justification was the same as for the first war: Rwanda wanted to eliminate the Hutu extremists who were hiding in Congo. But the larger objective, obvious by the deployment and strategy of the invading forces, was forcing regime change in Kinshasa for the second time in two years.

But unlike the First Congo War, when the rest of Africa and the West were prepared to turn a blind eye to the aggression in order to be rid of Mobutu, the conflict drew in foreign powers that backed Kabila. He secured crucial military help from Angola and Zimbabwe and to a lesser extent from Namibia, Chad, and Libya.

Nine different countries fought each other to a stalemate. The conflict split Congo roughly into three parts. The western third was under the control of forces loyal to Kabila, the north was run by Uganda-backed rebels, and the east, including Bukavu, was occupied by Rwanda and its proxies.

We began our work at Panzi against the ominous and frightening backdrop of the start of the Second Congo War. Bukavu teemed with regular Rwandan forces, and the province was administered by the RCD, a ragtag bunch of intellectuals and former officials put together by Rwanda.

Our plans soon went awry. Our tents and operating material were looted from a UNICEF warehouse in the early stages of the fighting. Our plan B was to renovate two small and nearly derelict buildings on a site in Panzi dating back to when the land had been a plantation. They were in a bad state: there was grass pushing out from between the stonework; parts of their roofs had collapsed; and the doors, window frames, and floors had been plundered.

But they were better than nothing. Without the tents, we needed to start somewhere. We worked on sourcing building materials to renovate them. We started the process again of securing medical supplies and equipment, which were in short supply.

In September 1999, three years after leaving Lemera at the start of the First Congo War and a year after the beginning of the next, I was at the site when our first patient arrived and I heard those familiar and fateful words: "You're needed, Doctor, right away. It's an emergency."

Our very first patient, I eventually learned, had been a victim of gang rape by Rwandan soldiers.

She spent several months with us recovering from her injuries. She never told me the full story herself, but I learned about what had happened to her from one of her relatives.

She had been at home when five soldiers had come to the door. She had refused to open up, so they barged in, pointing their weapons at her. They told her not to scream or they would shoot. They held her down and raped her. The last man, seeing the brutalized and semi-conscious body of his victim in front of him, had drawn his gun and shot her in the groin.

She still lives in Bukavu. We managed to save her leg, and the bullet missed her reproductive system, but she limps to this day. It was a heinous crime, but it was far from an isolated case.

In the first three months of work at Panzi, from September to December 1999, our hospital records show that we had forty-five women arrive with injuries inflicted during rape. There was no time to think about, let alone celebrate, the official opening of the hospital.

I had seen terrible wounds before when treating the injured in Lemera from the Hutu-Tutsi clashes over the border in Burundi and Rwanda. I knew that the capacity of man to inflict suffering on others had no bounds. But I was profoundly affected by what I witnessed. The nature of the rape injuries, and their frequency, was unprecedented.

There had been rapes before this time, of course. Sexual violence was a reality in Congo, as it is in all societies where men hold the social and political power and women are treated as objects and inferior citizens. But Congolese men were no more dangerous than their counterparts elsewhere in Africa or indeed in the West. I want to stress this point because for years now Congo has been routinely referred to as the "rape capital of the world" in media reports, following an expression once used by a UN official. It is an unfortunate label that has stuck, one hundred years after my country became known as the "heart of darkness" thanks to Joseph Conrad's book of the same name.

During my travels abroad talking about my work, I have been asked whether there is something inherently violent and misogynistic about Congolese men that might explain the atrocities of the last two decades. Sometimes I sense echoes of racist assumptions that Black or African men are more sexually voracious than others, less able to restrain their impulses, or are more prone to violence. None of this is true.

Accounts of rape are as old as written history, while the last century is littered with conflicts containing horrifying sexual violence across all continents and cultures. Around the same time Congo descended into chaos, men and soldiers in the former Yugoslavia in Europe were systematically raping. There were mass rapes committed during World War II in the European and Asian zones of that conflict, as well as in Vietnam by American soldiers.

What has happened in Congo is singular insofar as it results from a particular context: a country with a sad history of ruthless exploitation, of misrule, of the gradual erosion of social structures and institutions, and then decades of war and conflict. It is also universal, because the underlying explanations of sexual violence are relevant everywhere, in times of both war and peace.

In the first years of work at Panzi, each time we admitted a new injured woman it would affect me terribly. Once we'd operated and the patient was recovering, I would sit down next to the bed and ask her to explain what had happened. Trying to understand my patients' suffering seemed like part of my duty. I listened and did my best to empathize. I also needed to understand the injuries I was seeing.

Some would make up stories—that they had slipped and impaled themselves on something. Others made it clear they'd rather not talk or declined to give the full picture, like our first patient. But many opened up about their experiences, which were all different but had many things in common.

Most of the women we treated at the beginning came from Bukavu and the surrounding villages. They had all been raped by armed men—soldiers or rebels. Sometimes they were in their homes, while at other times they had been out in the fields working, or they had been snatched while walking to do the washing in a local stream or fetching water or charcoal.

Many of them had injuries inflicted with extreme violence. Some had been shot deliberately in their genitals. The rapists would insert their guns into a victim's vagina and then press the trigger. Others had had sticks, sharp objects, or burning plastic forced inside them. One woman had been forced to squat over a barbecue fire, causing her grievous burns.

They were frequently raped in front of their husbands, sometimes in front of their children. Children were occasionally forced to join in—under pain of death.

I would listen and try to offer comfort. Sometimes the patient would stare blankly as they put words to the scarcely imaginable acts they had suffered, the sentences falling weakly from their lips as if they were describing a distant scene.

Others would turn away and cover their eyes with their hands, as if in a physical struggle with torment they could not banish from their minds. Some shook with sobs that came in great physical heaves; others cried quietly, dark wet lines forming down their cheeks.

Many uttered the same desperate expression: "They've killed me."

I noticed how many women had a feeling of being detached from their own bodies, as if their attackers had severed some vital link between their sense of self and their physical existence. Over time, we would come to understand this condition as "dissociation"—a common reaction to trauma. Some patients would describe feeling as if their spirit had left their body.

Sexual abuse creates deep psychological wounds and is processed differently from other types of physical assault. Sexual violence is an attack on our most private parts. Not having control over our genitals creates a deep mental disturbance and sense of humiliation that every torturer understands.

The sense of violation often also leads to a profound loss of confidence in one's fellow human beings, as if the most basic rule of our common existence—that we will avoid inflicting wanton suffering on each other—has been broken. As they lay in their beds, my patients would wonder aloud why their attacker had acted so cruelly, unmoved by their pain and screams.

After returning from France, at Lemera, I became adept at treating obstetric fistulas—the openings that can form between the vagina and the bladder, or the vagina and the rectum, during obstructed labor. In Panzi, I was treating fistulas on a regular basis, caused deliberately by men, as well as performing cosmetic surgery in order to try to restore my patients' sense of self.

Because of my expertise, we became the regional center for treatment. Complicated cases were brought to us from all over the province. In our first full year of operation, in 2000, I operated on 135 women. Thereafter the figures began to grow exponentially. By 2004–2005, we were treating 3,000 women annually. And this was just the tip of the iceberg.

Estimating the number of rapes in Congo is fraught with difficulty because of the lack of reliable data and the reluctance of women to report crimes against them. One widely cited study by US researchers in 2011, using Congolese survey data, estimated that more than four hundred thousand women were raped in Congo every year.[2] Doubts have been raised about its methodology, though the figure does not seem wildly unrealistic to me. There are atrocities that see every woman and girl of a whole village raped in the same evening, which can mean two hundred new victims in the space of a few hours.

The only data we can trust with certainty are hospital admissions. Panzi has treated around sixty thousand survivors of sexual violence since its opening. The only other hospital equipped to treat rape injuries in the region is in Goma, HEAL Africa. It has treated around thirty thousand women.

But these figures count only the most serious cases: women requiring surgery or sophisticated medical care. For every victim who makes it to a hospital, how many others suffer in silence or never seek treatment? We will probably never know.

Lying in bed at night in the early years, I would often feel my throat tightening and a weight descend on my shoulders and body, as if the air had grown denser around me. I would play over the same heartbreaking questions I fielded again and again from patients: Will I fully recover? Will I be able to have children? Will I ever be able to have sex again? In so many cases, the answer was no.

I've had various periods in my life when I have struggled to get enough sleep. When we started work at Panzi, some nights I would fail to shut my eyes for more than a couple of hours. I tossed and turned in bed. I stared up in the silent darkness of the room, feeling oppressed by the pitch black. I imagined the physical struggles, the fears, and the screams of my patients.

My restlessness would sometimes wake up Madeleine, who would try to comfort me. She was working at the hospital at that time as an assistant radiologist, so she was aware of the cases we were seeing. Sometimes we'd talk in the evenings about our work, but generally we tried to separate it from our home life. Often this was impossible given the stresses we were all under.

It had an impact on our family life, of course. I grew worried about security, particularly about the safety of Madeleine and my daughters. I became overprotective and sometimes suffocating for my children, whom I constantly worried about. I'd be at work and suddenly feel compelled to call home and check on where they were and what they were doing.

I also became a nervous perfectionist during surgery, trying to do everything within my power to repair the damage wrought on my patients' bodies. All good surgeons should push themselves to improve. But if the drive for excellence becomes obsessive, it can be counterproductive.

I'd ask, What will her life be like after this? over and over again in my head as I worked. An operation that should have taken me two hours was suddenly taking four. It was tiring for the rest of the surgical team and I was causing major disruption to the hospital timetables.

And I began wondering how much I was helping the women

themselves. I'd often cry with them. Men who are unable to cry are often the most dangerous ones, I've found. But I wasn't sure I was doing the right thing.

Patients looked to me for reassurance. If I was crying, their doctor, did that mean their injuries were particularly severe and their chances of recovery slim? Was their story worse than everyone else's? Perhaps they questioned whether I was able to do my job in such an unstable emotional state.

It was obvious that we needed to be better at providing support to help victims deal with their trauma. And I needed to look after myself better. I couldn't be the medical director of the hospital, a surgeon, and a psychologist. The psychological care needed to be handled by a specialized team.

Starting around 2001, we put in place a new system. There were no clinical psychologists in the region, but we found an occupational psychologist who was willing to move from the business sector to the medical one. And we trained up some of the more experienced women among the nursing staff. What they lacked in formal education they made up for with compassion, experience, and a willingness to listen.

Each new patient was invited to meet the psychological support team and was assessed for symptoms of trauma. Over time, our techniques have become more sophisticated. We've since had help from clinicians from the United States, Canada, and Europe.

Every woman who comes to the hospital with rape injuries is also assigned to someone in our team of *mamans chéries,* or "loving moms." They have no equivalent in other hospitals: they are part nurse, part social worker, part psychologist.

They are amazing women, full of warmth and vitality, who act as confidantes and guides. They administer hugs and music as much as medicine. And they are moms in the real sense: they help our patients emerge from their torpor, assisting with a sort of rebirth, both physical and psychological.

Each patient is assessed and her behavior classified according to whether she shows symptoms of severe, mild, or an absence of trauma. Severe cases are immediately referred to one of our psychiatrists for follow-up.

This is an attempt to classify the responses of patients and prioritize our resources, because all victims of sexual abuse react differently. Each incident is experienced in a unique way depending on the circumstances, the degree of violence used, and the identity of the perpetrator or perpetrators. There is a whole spectrum of reactions. There is no "normal," and an absence of trauma does not mitigate the seriousness of the crime.

Our approach has always been "survivor centered," even though we didn't call it this at the beginning. It means that we treat each case individually and recognize that there is no one-size-fits-all approach to dealing with the consequences of sexual violence. The psychological care process is driven by what the patient identifies as her needs.

Some women develop a visceral aversion to all men, particularly anyone who reminds them of their attacker. The sight of a soldier in uniform or a machine gun can trigger an involuntary flashback and physical reaction. Rape can frequently result in hyposexuality—a lack of interest and rejection of sex—or its opposite, hypersexuality. Because victims can feel dissociated from their bodies, which they may no longer value, sometimes they enter into inappropriate sexual relations.

Many experience shame, self-loathing, and guilt afterward. These are common but not universal feelings. The impact of trauma must be understood as diverse and varied. Some women may not feel or show any symptoms of their trauma in the immediate aftermath.

Understanding my patients' needs and improving our methods has been a journey for me. At each step, I have understood more and more about how sexual assault is experienced and the best ways of encouraging the healing process.

My career changed course again with the opening of Panzi Hospital. As a young doctor, I had started out thinking I was going to be a pediatrician but had switched to focus on maternal health after seeing the lack of care for women during pregnancy and childbirth in Lemera. Now I was changing again, owing to events beyond my control, to become a specialist in treating rape injuries.

At various points, particularly at the beginning but not only then, I have doubted whether I could carry on. I've felt my work crush my spirit, sadness descend on me like a shroud. It has sometimes shaken my faith in my fellow human beings. There is only so much anyone can take of witnessing bodies, lives, and communities being torn apart.

I was able to carry on only because of my patients. My decision to become a obstetrician-gynecologist had been motivated by the admiration I felt for the women of Lemera, for their strength and forbearance as they limped to the hospital, for their power in childbirth. As well as wanting to tackle the injustice of their lives, and a society that neither valued them nor celebrated their achievements, I was drawn forward and inspired by the displays of resilience I witnessed.

The same thing happened at Panzi in different circumstances. I felt in awe of the vitality and power of the women I treated.

It was different with the men. We have admitted many male rape victims over the years, but they are a minority, as they are globally among victims of sexual violence. Often they have been sodomized or abused publicly or in front of their families.

As patients, they have often seemed more difficult to help. The humiliation seems to have pulverized their masculinity, their sense of self, their control and ability to protect themselves and others. In my experience, male patients find it far harder to recover from the immediate aftermath of a sexual assault and begin a new life. Addictions often follow, and suicide is an all-too-common tragic end.

I remember the case of a man in 2008 who was admitted for care at the hospital after his penis had been cut off. First, I was surprised at how much attention he received in the media. His photo was published in the Congolese newspapers and his story was even written up overseas. I had treated literally hundreds of female patients whose genitals had been mutilated but who did not generate a fraction of the interest.

This particular man was almost impossible to care for. He was suffering from such severe mental health problems that I couldn't get through to him to explain how he would need to learn to live with his handicap. Yet the women I treated, even those whose vaginas were destroyed by their attackers, who faced a life without children or sex, managed in the most part to find reasons to live. They continued to fight. They managed to find a sense of new meaning for their existence.

I drew my strength from them. If they could find the desire and courage to carry on, then I had to keep my faith and my concentration in order to help provide them with the future they so ardently desired for themselves.

I want to tell you about a woman from this early era of Panzi who exemplifies resilience. She's one of many who have inspired me to keep going on the mornings when I would get out of bed feeling groggy after another sleepless night. What she taught me about inner strength is a lesson to us all. Let's call her Bernadette.

She is from the region of Fizi to the south of Bukavu. Her father was the *mwami,* or local chief, who had four wives in total. Bernadette was one of his more than fifteen children, but her mother fell out of favor and was sent away when Bernadette was only eight. "As a child, I didn't ever go hungry. The thing I missed out on was affection," she told me in one of our many conversations.

She remembers her father having visitors constantly. People would come to see him whenever there was a dispute in the village, between neighbors over land or between families over marriages, crime, or inheritance. Her father would call meetings and mediate. He would also allocate land to newcomers and give permission for new buildings, such as churches, just as the *mwami* does in my village.

At sixteen, Bernadette fell pregnant to her French-language tutor, a man five years older than she was. She didn't love him, but she felt obliged to wed. He paid her dowry and a marriage was arranged, opening a new period in her life that would contain no more tenderness than her childhood. Three times she fell pregnant to him, three times her child was stillborn.

When the Second Congo War came in 1998, because of tensions with her in-laws, Bernadette moved out of her marital home and back to her own family. Her father refused to leave the village as others fled for safety. "If I'm going to die, I prefer to die here," he told her.

There was a camp of Rwandan soldiers stationed in the village. Every so often it would be attacked. "We lived in fear all the time," Bernadette remembered.

In her early twenties, she was walking along a path in the forest a few miles outside the village. She was with an older woman who worked for her family. The path was quiet and shaded, with the noise of a river rushing next to them. She felt vulnerable, and normally she would have avoided being there, but she was going to see an older brother whose wife had died.

"Stop," she heard.

A group of Rwandan soldiers from the camp in her village emerged from the undergrowth. They were young, in uniform, and armed. Bernadette wanted to run but did her best to stay calm. She knew she was in danger.

One of them ordered the older woman away but said Bernadette had to stay to carry him across the river, an impossible task given the depth of the water and mismatch in size.

As soon as the older woman had left, Bernadette braced herself. The man who had spoken, who seemed to be the leader of the group, grabbed her by the arm and began dragging her into the trees. Others started tearing at her clothes. Bernadette screamed for help and tried to fight them off. A local man walking along the path appeared briefly, glanced across, but scuttled away.

Bernadette continued to scream and struggle with them. The leader drew a knife and put it to her throat. Bernadette screamed some more. At the end, one of the group put his gun up to her vagina and fired off a round.

She remembers the deafening noise, the feeling of shock. But she continued to struggle, as blood drenched her *pagne* from the waist down. Her attackers ran off.

Bernadette's older walking companion had been waiting nearby, too scared to return, but when she heard the gunshot she ran back to investigate. She found Bernadette collapsed in a heap where the soldier had left her.

Together, with Bernadette leaning on the older woman for support, they limped to the local village, agonizing step by step. The pain was so overwhelming that Bernadette feared she would lose consciousness and never make it. She was taken to a local hospital, where she received a blood transfusion, then she was transferred to Panzi.

We operated on her four times. She also traveled to Addis Adaba for care for her fistula, which required another four interventions. But though her body recovered, her life was changed forever. Her husband abandoned her definitively afterward. He never called during her long recovery.

After everything she had been through, it might have been difficult to find meaning in her life. Her marriage and hopes for a family of her own were dashed. Members of her own family treated her as cursed and an embarrassment. Yet she showed a determination to rebuild in Bukavu every bit as impressive as her bravery in fighting with her attackers.

She completed three years of high school education in her twenties, earning her state diploma, then began studying at a nursing college, rekindling an interest she had felt as a child. "After everything I've been through, all the help I've received, I wanted to do something for others," she decided.

She couldn't afford to take the bus to college, so she walked for an hour and a half each way from her home, weaving through traffic and keeping her balance on the slippery mud tracks of Bukavu. She did this for four years, showing a single-mindedness and quiet determination that are her hallmarks.

Bernadette specialized further as an anesthetist and is now working at Panzi Hospital. When I asked her to explain her choice, she was adamant. "I know what pain is," she said. "I remember my walk back to the village from the forest. You can't imagine the torture. I remember the feeling of waking up after every operation I've had here. I don't want others to feel that agony."

Each working day she spends hours in surgery, literally taking away the pain of other women. Before and after, she works with survivors during physiotherapy sessions, helping them regain muscle strength and their continence. And in between sessions, she gives encouragement, she shares her own story, she helps others believe in their futures through the power of her example.

Women like Bernadette have to rely on extraordinary inner reserves of resilience because our society treats them almost as callously as their aggressors. When my patients tell me, "They've killed me," when they wake from surgery or lie recovering in the wards, what they mean is that part of them has died—but also that they are dead in the eyes of people around them, loved ones and family members.

Almost none of the married women in the wards of Panzi have visits from their husbands. Most find themselves rejected and divorced afterward. Once violated, they are seen as soiled. They are often viewed as being somehow responsible for their own abuse, having invited an attack through their behavior. I've known cases of women condemned by their own church leaders for adultery and the "sin" of being raped.

When a woman is treated as a possession, passed from father to husband at the time of marriage, they can be cast aside in favor of a new one. Wives find themselves ejected from the family home. It is even worse if they have fallen pregnant from the attack.

I suspect, deep down, that a raped wife is seen by men as a reminder of their own failure to perform what they see as their fundamental duty to protect. They prefer to banish this source of suffering rather than question it or see it as a challenge to be overcome as a couple. Sometimes the sisters and mother of a husband will help him find a new partner.

The isolation and stigmatization of victims does not end there. Often a victim will be rejected by her own parents and then ostracized by her community. Again, the impulse is to banish something seen as shameful and embarrassing rather than deal with it. This often results in taunts and insults, but also exclusion from the vital collective work of farming in villages, which relies on groups doing the sowing and harvesting together.

If the victim is suffering from a fistula caused by rape, the consequences are even more severe because of the personal hygiene problems associated with this condition.

Once marginalized, forced to live alone or with only their children as company, raped women are then preyed on by other men, who see them as promiscuous and easy targets. In the worst cases, the psychological distress caused by this treatment can lead survivors to be condemned as "bad spirits" or witches, which sometimes results in them being chased away or murdered.

This pattern can be observed across the world, sadly, wherever women are seen as possessions and where their value is measured by their "honor." You see it in the strict patriarchal conventions of tribal groups in Pakistan and the traditions that govern villages in rural India. The so-called honor killings of women there are intended to purge communities of the shame and sin of sexual assault. They pile injustice upon injustice.

Victim blaming takes on different forms but is still rife in all countries. In the West, the same traditions—the focus on "honor" as exemplified by virginity and chastity—dominated until relatively recently. The overwhelming majority of women in Western countries do not report sexual assaults, largely out of fear of how they will be viewed. Those who do routinely have their motives and behavior questioned. They are suspected of having contributed to or somehow encouraged sexual abuse, through their behavior or their way of dressing.

This bias can be seen in the way cases are reported in the media and treated by the criminal justice system.

Toronto police officer Michael Sanguinetti became infamous for victim blaming during a presentation to students in 2011 on college campus safety after he advised that "women should avoid dressing like sluts in order not to be victimized." Sanguinetti might think he had little in common with the average Congolese husband, being separated by seven thousand miles and a gulf in living standards, language, and culture. Yet they both view raped women as being responsible for their own assaults.

Sanguinetti's speech sparked the SlutWalk movement founded by two Canadian students in response to his so-called advice. It brought women onto the streets in hundreds of cities around the world, many of them dressing provocatively to make a statement. I followed the debate among feminists afterward about whether there was a need to reclaim the word "slut"—a misogynistic insult with no equivalent for promiscuous men, of course—and the decision by many protesters to appear in lingerie or high heels.

Whatever the means, the message was that attitudes needed to change. This is vital work. All societies need to shift the blame, the guilt, and the responsibility for sexual violence from women onto their abusers. The perpetrator needs to pay the price, not the victim.

Different countries and cultures are further along than others, but none has reached a point where survivors of sexual violence can expect to be treated with sympathy and offered unconditional support by everyone from community leaders to police officers, judges, journalists, politicians, and their own families.

In our early work at the start of the century, the stigmatization of survivors was so strong in Congo that I felt we needed to go much further with our ambitions for the hospital. Medically, we were improving all the time. I was becoming more and more adept at operating on fistulas. Our psychological care programs developed with limited resources. But we weren't doing enough.

I've always said to myself that emotion without action is pointless. It's a mantra I live by. We must all find ways of channeling our feelings of sadness, disgust, admiration, and love into decisions that help reduce the suffering of others.

I knew I needed to find an opposite reaction to the unleashing of so much hatred and depravity in eastern Congo. The only possible response was to love more and spread it more widely. We needed to improve, expand, reach more people, help rebuild more lives, and call out the cruel social conventions that affected survivors. Inspirational women such as Bernadette showed what could be achieved.

She gives the same advice to all of the survivors who seek her out. "It's not the end of their lives, there's another life waiting if they want it. Their injuries, the rape, the memories, they won't go away. You have to accept them. We can't wish them away, however much we'd like to. But with one foot in front of the other, every day, slowly, over time, we can leave them behind."

Instead of abandoning her, Bernadette's family has embraced her as a heroine. She looks after several of her nieces and nephews at her home in Bukavu. And she smiles with pride every time she recalls how many Bernadettes have been born after her. Several of her brothers and sisters have named their children in her honor.

4

PAIN AND POWER

*W*amuzila first came to the hospital in 2002. She was a delicate girl with fine features. Around seventeen at the time, she was a spirited character who held her own in discussions with others much older than her. Her almond-shaped eyes sparkled with life and kindness but also contained traces of great sadness and innocence lost.

She was from the Shabunda region, around 160 miles to the west of Bukavu. That doesn't sound far, but to reach it one must cross the mountains and descend into the flatness and humidity of dense tropical rain forest. There is no road connection, and only the brave or heavily protected would attempt to reach it overland. Access is by plane only, using a small jungle airstrip when the weather is fair. It may as well be a different country, such is its isolation.

Shabunda is an enclave, ringed at its extremities by hills that form the edge of the floodplain of the river Ulindi, which empties into the mighty Congo to the north. It has little electricity or piped water. Its villages, dirt roads, and mines are all scattered around the valley.

Wamuzila had no formal education, a common affliction for girls like her in rural areas. If there is a local school, many parents will send only their sons for a few years, just enough so they can learn to read and write.

It's hard to get a reliable estimate of literacy levels in Congo because of poor data collection by the government and the fact that large portions of the country are no-go areas because of rebel groups. Primary school is obligatory and free for all in theory. But girls and women are the ones who overwhelmingly miss out.

An estimate in 2016 from UNESCO, the UN's education and cultural agency, was that one in three Congolese women was illiterate, compared with one in ten men.[1] This figure seems an underestimate to me; one need only travel to villages thirty minutes outside of Bukavu to witness the depth of the problem. Worldwide, there are an estimated 750 million adults unable to read or write a simple sentence. Most of them are women in Africa or South Asia.

Life in Shabunda is hard and precarious. In its humid climate, clouds of mosquitoes spread malaria, the biggest killer locally. The rivers and streams contain a host of waterborne diseases, making diarrhea another major cause of mortality, particularly for children and the elderly. Families are large; resources are spread thin.

Wamuzila spent her childhood as millions of other girls like her do, as an extra pair of hands in the daily struggle of subsistence farming. She knew how to grow cassava, rice, and corn, how to extract oil from the greasy red seeds of the palm tree, or when to pick peanuts or bananas. She knew the texture and heaviness of the rich and fertile soil in the fields around her village. She learned to farm, expecting that, probably in her midteens, she would marry, then bear children and provide for her own family.

She grew up knowing little about the outside world, but this changed in the mid-1990s. When rebels and Rwandan forces invaded Congo in 1996 at the start of the First Congo War, tens of thousands of Hutu refugees from the camps around Bukavu and along the Congo-Rwanda border fled inland toward places such as Shabunda. They were pursued by Rwandan forces. Thousands were bludgeoned to death, bayoneted, or locked in houses that were set on fire. Locals were pressed into action to dig mass graves.

In one incident in February 1997, around five hundred people were massacred by rebels and the Rwandan army at a bridge over the Ulindi River, a few miles from the main town in the region. After the massacre, villagers were made to dump the bodies in the river and clean the bridge.[2]

The Hutu extremists responsible for the genocide found the terrain and thick forest of Shabunda ideal as a place to hide. They led their families deep into the jungle and set up camps where they could evade detection. They formed a militia, called the Democratic Forces for the Liberation of Rwanda (FDLR).

In the Second Congo War, starting in August 1998, there were more clashes between the invading Rwandan armed forces and the Hutu rebels around Shabunda. Kabila began dropping arms and supplies for the Hutu. As the violence spiraled, Congolese militias called Mai-Mai sprang up to defend the local population against the continuation of the Rwandan ethnic war on Congolese soil.

Civilians found themselves in the crossfire between the warring parties; many were massacred, supposedly for offering support to one side or the other. Over time, the Mai-Mai groups became just as predatory as the foreign forces they were meant to be guarding against.

Wamuzila's tough but quiet childhood was turned upside down. The FDLR militia terrorized the Shabunda region. Its foot soldiers would leave their jungle camps and turn up in villages in dirty civilian clothes, AK-47s slung over their shoulders. They were distinguishable from the Rwandan armed forces, who wore crisp military fatigues and rubber boots.

The rebels would ask the locals to hand over supplies—food or medicine—as well as boys and young men who would be taken away as new recruits. Because of the plundering, farming became even harder. Malnutrition rose. Livestock became scarce, but the price of goats or chickens actually fell: no one wanted to buy them because they knew they would be instantly stolen.

If a village resisted, it would be attacked. Houses would be burned, men shot, and women raped in public. The rebels used this brutality to send a message to other communities that might think about standing up for themselves. A whole settlement might be torched if its population was suspected of helping "the enemy," which could be anyone from the Rwandan army to a rival militia.

From the beginning, the militiamen deliberately targeted women and girls. During the day, they would be snatched as they walked on forest tracks. Women developed strategies to try to keep safe, such as staying in groups or only sending older women out for errands on their own, on the assumption that they were less vulnerable to kidnap and rape. At night, groups of fighters three to four strong would go house to house looking for prey. Fathers or husbands who tried to put up a fight to defend their wife or daughters were killed on the spot.

Young, pretty, and unmarried girls were spared immediate death. They were marched away from their homes into the jungle at gunpoint. From then on, they were kept as slaves by pitiless masters, their physical and mental health ground down slowly, blow by blow, chipped away over weeks and sometimes months of abuse, leaving them so low and desperate that they felt envious of family members who had died suddenly from bullets or machete blows.

Wamuzila was seized in her village at night during an attack by the FDLR in 2001. Only slightly built, she thrashed her arms at first and squirmed her teenage body with all her force against the weight of the drunken brutes who pinned her down and raped her. Then they led her into the forest.

She cried and pleaded with her attackers to let her go as she limped along the muddy paths in pitch darkness, distraught but still hoping they would take pity on her. They barked at her to keep walking.

Once they reached their base camp, they tied her to a tree like an animal. From then on, at any time, when sober during the day or drunk on palm wine and aggressive at night, members of the militia visited to force themselves on her. The camp moved regularly, the fighters never staying in the same place for more than a few weeks in one spot.

She spent nearly a year like this. She was fed rotten food or leftovers and slept out in the open, shivering at night under leaves and branches. She was frequently sick and almost always in pain from injuries and infections inflicted by her tormentors.

Falling pregnant to her attackers eventually brought an end to the torture. She was released, not out of sympathy, of course. There is no heroic figure in her story who found a conscience or felt compassion for her. She was simply no longer of any use as a sex slave.

She tried to give birth in the camp, on the ground in the middle of a forest: a teenager facing the moment alone. She remembered thinking she was going to die from the pain, which felt even worse than anything else she had experienced up until then. She couldn't expel the baby. The head was stuck.

Her captors moved on and abandoned her. But her desire to live was so extraordinarily powerful that she was able to struggle to her feet. Despite everything she had lived through, she found the strength to stumble through the undergrowth, the fetus still stuck in her abdomen, until she saw smoke in the distance. She walked toward it and into a village where people took fright. She managed to mumble a few words in her language, Kirega, before collapsing.

Her baby died, and once shrunken inside her, she was finally able to eject its lifeless form. The obstructed labor caused damage to her genitals and resulted in two different fistulas, one between her rectum and vagina and another between her bladder and vagina. Two weeks after leaving the forest, she was found by staff of Médecins Sans Frontières (MSF; Doctors Without Borders), the medical aid group.

They called our hospital and asked if we could admit her. She was brought from Shabunda, like so many other victims before and since then, aboard a small plane chartered by the organization.

She arrived conscious but seriously ill, in excruciating pain, and with the telltale odor of fistula patients. She was like an injured bird, a small crumpled creature, weak and vulnerable.

The extent of her injuries and age made her a complicated case, but sadly not an unusual one. The first step is always to clean up the patient and examine her injuries. Fluids, pain relief, and antibiotics are administered if needed. We screen for sexually transmitted diseases and HIV as a matter of course. We run blood tests to check hemoglobin levels. Many women arrive suffering from anemia due to malnutrition.

In total, Wamuzila required four operations. I led them all myself.

In the first one we fitted a colostomy bag, a relatively simple procedure in which a small incision is made in the abdomen through which the colon can be brought out. This prevents fecal matter causing infection to internal injuries.

The second operation tackled the vesicovaginal fistula—the hole between her bladder and her vagina. I remember we were in the theater for three or four hours, from early in the morning until lunchtime. It is always a complicated procedure, with the level of difficulty determined by the size and, above all, the location of the lesions.

I owe a debt of gratitude to two people in particular for my expertise in treating fistulas, both of whom demonstrated generosity and grace in sharing their knowledge with me. The first is Catherine Hamlin, a remarkable Australian woman who founded the Addis Ababa Fistula Hospital in 1974 with her husband, Reginald.

Over their careers, the Hamlins treated tens of thousands of women. I had the honor of training briefly with Catherine after my time in France. Then in her midseventies, she operated and taught with the vigor and passion of a person half her age. She retained the same dedication to women in Africa right up to her death in 2020 at the age of ninety-six.

The second teacher is my dear friend Guy-Bernard Cadière, a Belgian surgeon and steadfast supporter of Panzi Hospital, who trained me in noninvasive keyhole surgery techniques using a laparoscope. No one ever succeeds alone, and remembering our teachers and forerunners is a useful exercise in humility.

The original pioneer in my specialized field of medicine is not a man I recollect with affection, however.

The first-ever successful treatment of a fistula is credited to an individual often described as the "father of gynecology," an American doctor by the name of James Marion Sims who practiced in

Alabama in the mid-1800s. He was also behind the design of the speculum still used today, the device used to open up the vaginal walls, and the so-called Sims position for examinations.

As students, we learned of him in our textbooks and were taught about his techniques. One could not help being impressed by this distant figure whose influence over our training continued so strongly even a century after his death. I discovered the full story of his life and methods only much later. All African and Black gynecologists have reason in particular to feel uneasy about his legacy.

While taking part at a conference on fistulas in Boston in 2008, I heard a Black American anesthetist denounce his work in a remarkable presentation that silenced the room. She spoke passionately and angrily about how Sims had conducted all of his experimental work treating fistulas on slaves without giving them anesthesia. One of them, called Anarcha, he operated on more than thirty times.

The revelation spurred me to read more on his history. Although he still has defenders within my profession—who argue that he found a solution for a previously incurable condition—his record has since been rightly reassessed. A large bronze statue of him was removed from Central Park in New York City in 2018.

Though his contributions in the medical field are unquestioned, whenever I envisage him, I see his forgotten patients surrounding him—Anarcha and other women he names in his writings, such as Lucy and Betsey. They are true heroines without whom Sims would not have won fame and fortune.

In rare fistula cases, for around one in fifty women I operate on in Panzi, we need to resort to reconstructive surgery based on a technique named after the German gynecologist Heinrich Martius, who first described it in 1928. This is for large fistulas or when previous surgery has failed. It entails cutting a flap of subcutaneous fat from the pelvic area or the bulbocavernosus muscle and using this to cover and plug the tear.

Wamuzila recovered well from the first two rounds of surgery, and after three months we were ready to repair the remaining recto-vaginal fistula. The difficulty of this procedure again depends on the location, whether the injury is in the lower, middle, or upper part of the vagina. The deeper the injury, the more difficult it is to access. Often the procedure must start with reconstruction of the sphincter, which can be damaged in cases of birth-related and traumatic fistulas.

Wamuzila stayed with us for around six months. The final round of surgery entailed removing the colostomy bag and reconnecting the colon. By the end, her wounds had healed completely. She was walking around without discomfort. She had renewed control over her bladder and bowels.

The length of her stay meant she made friends in the hospital with fellow patients and staff. She sang enthusiastically at the church service we hold every morning at seven A.M. in the courtyard just outside my office. I would watch her taking part, knowing her cruel history and marveling at her recovery, as I paused to take a few minutes to breathe in the prayer and music myself, my morning ritual before starting work.

As part of a small-scale vocational training program we had running at that time, Wamuzila learned how to make soap from palm oil, the idea being that she could start a small business when she returned home.

It became time to think about her returning to her village. We had a limited number of beds and the needs were huge. We'd have new rape victims arriving every day that needed attention.

We contacted MSF. They had an aircraft returning to Shabunda in the next few days and agreed to hold a place for Wamuzila.

The news filled her with fear. She knew there would be no warm homecoming after around eighteen months away. The night before her scheduled departure, she began crying and begged the nurses to let her stay.

"I don't want to go back," she said, sobbing. "I'm happy here in the hospital, I'm looked after. When I go home, everyone will point at me and make fun of me." It was heartbreaking to hear about, but we were in an impossible situation.

The following morning, when the MSF vehicle arrived to take her to the airport, I went to see her on the ward to say goodbye. We'd chatted a lot during her stay. She used to call me "papa" as we talked about her childhood and fears for the future.

She'd confided in me about her feelings of shame for having lost her virginity to her attackers. I'd explained, as I did to all my young patients, that virginity can never be taken; it can only be relinquished freely. I'd repeat over and over again how the only shame and dishonor were for her rapists, not her.

When I told her the car would be arriving soon, she refused to go outside. Then she began crying again, demanding to stay at the hospital. I tried to reason with her; I explained the constraints. But she grew hysterical. She threw herself on the floor, her body went limp, and she refused to stand. She screwed her eyes shut and screamed that she was sick and shouldn't go back.

To calm her down, we agreed to let her stay so that we could examine her. The car was sent away and the plane left that day without her. The nurses checked her parameters, which were normal. There was no sign of any illness.

Her evident suffering underlined to me just how much our patients, once they left the safety and supportive environment of the hospital, faced a new set of obstacles. At Panzi, they were listened to and cared for by our medics but also our *mamans chéries*. Their injuries did not revolt anyone. For girls like Wamuzila, ours was perhaps the only environment they had ever known where they felt loved and supported.

But the outside world was hostile. Once home, they knew they would be viewed not as people worthy of sympathy and support but as outsiders who brought disgrace and even bad luck.

Wamuzila was far from alone in reacting like this, but she was someone who made a big impact on me. As their discharge dates approached, we noticed other patients would begin reporting new health problems: pains in a different part of their bodies or breathing difficulties. It was impossible to know what was real or psychosomatic. The result was that we were having more and more difficulty freeing up beds.

Two weeks after the first scheduled departure date, MSF organized another transfer for Wamuzila and this time she agreed to leave. We hugged each other in front of the car. She was wearing a new set of clothes, which we provide for each discharged patient, and holding a bag of other going-home gifts: basins and goblets for making soap, plates, biscuits, and water for the journey.

There were more tears. She left heavyhearted, waving and smiling weakly from the backseat. I felt a tug of remorse and shame at my own powerlessness.

She forced me to reflect further on the nature of the injuries we were seeing at Panzi and the way we were caring for our patients. I felt in awe of Wamuzila and women like her. How anyone could fail to admire the resilience and bravery she demonstrated by returning home was beyond me. She was back on her feet, still capable of laughter and love. She hadn't been broken.

She was terrified of returning home because she knew she had fallen even further on the slippery social ladder in her village. She was right to apprehend the reception she would get back home.

We had achieved only a fraction of what was needed to truly lift her back up. She helped me see how we needed to go beyond simply treating injuries and trauma. We needed to engage in a cultural battle: against prejudice, bigotry, and exclusion. We needed to educate and encourage social change so that survivors of sexual violence felt that they had opportunities, that being raped was not a life sentence, that they could overcome the stigmatization they suffered from.

Doing all of this would require money. And managing the finances of the hospital had been difficult from the start.

We had expanded from our humble beginnings in our renovated former plantation buildings. Thanks to funding from several Swedish church and humanitarian groups, as well as the Swedish International Development Cooperation Agency, we were able to construct new purpose-built facilities: a dozen separate rectangular-shaped buildings, all one story high, set around courtyards where we planted palms, lawns, and flowers. They were all linked by concrete pathways, covered by tin roofs that provided shelter from the sun and rain. Along the sides of the pathways we planted roses and other flowers. By 2002, we had 125 beds.

We have since welcomed financial support from a number of aid groups and governments, including the United States Agency for International Development and the US-based nonprofits EngenderHealth and the Fistula Foundation. The British government also made a vital contribution, enabling us to open a wing in 2007 solely for survivors of sexual violence. We also rely on support from our Swedish church backers and receive annual funding from the European Union, which has stabilized our financial position. This means we no longer have to scramble throughout the year to bid for funding, with the attendant time-consuming forensic audits.

From time to time, we receive generous one-off donations of medical equipment from around the world. The hospital can sometimes seem like the buses and taxis that ply the streets of Bukavu: patched together with spare parts, some well worn, others new. It isn't the most efficient means of growing and requires constant management, but it is the only way we have been able to extend our services.

Either the Congolese state has been absent—in the early years, Bukavu was under rebel control—or it has been counterproductive when it has shown any interest.

Congo is often described as a "failed state," and any visitor cannot fail to observe the consequences. It can be heard in the voices of people who feel abandoned and neglected. It can be seen in the daily traffic chaos on our roads, the street crime, the unregulated construction, the pitch black that descends at nightfall because of the nonexistent public lighting.

Electricity and piped drinking water are luxuries enjoyed intermittently in Bukavu, if at all. Even children in middle-class homes are growing up washing in basins, without ever having had a shower or bath at home.

The budgets for the security forces are siphoned off, leaving a police force with barely any vehicles and no gasoline. Officers can often be seen hitching rides on motorbikes, a battered Kalashnikov slung over one shoulder. They depend on bribes for their wages and have to be paid to do tasks seen as the basic responsibility of officers in other countries.

Yet the state does exist. It lurks and pounces unpredictably, like a predator in the shadows. There are offices filled with badly paid bureaucrats, local and national officials, regulators and watchdogs, all ready to bring rules to bear when it suits them.

If the rules are unclear and opaque, if the bureaucracy is too thick to navigate, or if the security environment is too dangerous to operate in, all the better for raising your price. Paperwork and protection: both must be negotiated for a fee.

For many of these public servants, their job is not to serve and provide: it is to extract for personal gain. Some are malicious, others are simply doing their best to provide for their families in the only way they know how, muddling through like everyone else in Congo.

We have always been a nonprofit private hospital operated by a church organization, the Community of Pentecostal Churches in Central Africa. As one of a few facilities for the million-plus population of Bukavu, we should benefit from public funding for medication and equipment. In practice, we have never received anything from the state except for a few publicly funded doctors.

The lack of reliable electricity means we have to generate our own. Power cuts have been known to last three to four days. We receive only a few hours of electricity a day from the national grid at present, meaning we have two diesel engines running almost around the clock to power the incubators, ventilators, and other equipment that save lives daily.

The water supply at the beginning in 1999 was modest but just about sufficient for our needs. Over time it slowed to a trickle as more and more people moved to the Panzi area. We used to send a battered old water truck every day to fill up at the lake, but this eventually proved inadequate. In the end we built our own water pipeline, which runs for five miles from a water source in the hills behind Bukavu.

We run our own bus service for staff and patients because of the lack of public transport. We use our trucks and equipment to repair the roads nearby when they are blocked by landslides. And we need to be constantly on our toes to repel attempts at extortion.

I once had two officials from the local government present me with a bill of $30,000 for rain that we had collected from the roofs of the hospital. We store it in tanks and use it for cleaning purposes. All water was state property, they told me.

Another time, different officials arrived demanding taxes for the diesel that we stock on site for the generators. They brought with them a copy of legislation regulating gas stations and claimed it applied to us.

I refuse to pay bribes, but at other times the state has simply seized money from us. In 2014, I was given the Sakharov Prize by the European Parliament, an annual award for a human rights campaigner that comes with a check of fifty thousand euros. As with all the prize money I have ever won—including the Nobel Peace Prize—I had the check made out to the Panzi Foundation.

The day after the funds were deposited in Congo, our bank account was frozen by the local tax authority. We were unable to buy medication, and by the end of the month, we couldn't pay staff salaries. Our nurses and doctors went to demonstrate for the first time together outside the tax office in Bukavu.

I took on lawyers to fight the freeze. When the account was finally released, it was empty. European humanitarian money had been swallowed whole by an ever-hungry but hollow state. I never got the funds back.

In 2006, as awareness internationally flickered about the atrocities being committed in Congo, I was invited to New York City to address the United Nations. It was my first time in the United States and an opportunity, I hoped, to meet people who might be interested in supporting our work to put an end to the suffering of Congolese women.

The trip overall was dispiriting and made clear the depth of opposition in the Congolese government to publicly discussing the rape crisis at home. But it included a crucial encounter with someone who became a patron, a donor, and a personal friend. She would help us go beyond our initial, limited mission of patching up victims and returning them to their communities. She was someone who would help us serve women like Wamuzila much better.

After my speech at the UN, I was asked to take part in a public discussion at New York University on the issue of sexual violence. I was to be interviewed by Eve Ensler, the feminist playwright and creator of *The Vagina Monologues,* who has since changed her name to V. I confess to being slightly intimidated given V's fame and reputation.

The event was a revelation for me. It was the first time I had done this sort of interview, in public and in an English-speaking country. In V I found someone who both inspired me and made me feel instantly comfortable.

As I mentioned in my introduction, I spent years grappling with the idea of being a man promoting women's rights, suffering awkward silences or looks of incomprehension from both men and women when I talked about my work. With V it was different.

More than anyone at the time, she had worked to lift the shroud of embarrassment surrounding vaginas. She gave them a voice onstage in her play and she shared intimate stories about them. She educated and entertained people in a way I scarcely thought possible.

She was the first person I met who felt no shame in talking about the vagina publicly or her personal history of sexual violence at the hands of her father. We both shared the conviction that the reason vaginas were an object of so many taboos was so that men could continue to mistreat them behind closed doors.

Our event was a coming together of two minds from two very different worlds: a white Buddhist woman from New York and a Black Christian man from eastern Congo. She had rusty French, I had limited English at the time. I admired her ability to be at once so frank, so funny, and so committed. She appreciated my dedication as a man to fight against sexual violence.

We stayed in contact afterward and struck up a friendship. She was already a major funder of campaigns against violence against women across the world through her V-Day organization (the *V* stands for victory, valentine, and vagina), which she supported with the takings from *The Vagina Monologues* as it was staged around the world.

She had been apprehensive, too, about doing the event in New York, she told me afterward. She didn't know anything about me or much about Congo, but she felt she was going to learn things that would compel her to take action. That is one of the things I admire most about her: she acts on her emotions. She never thinks just words and sentiments are an appropriate response.

"Will you come to Congo?" I said as we parted in New York. "You'll always be welcome."

"I will. I'd love to," she replied immediately.

Less than a year later, she arrived.

As recognition of our work at Panzi has grown in recent years, I've received many famous guests from the worlds of entertainment and film. All of them have been moved by the stories they hear, but only a few show lasting commitment.

V was one of the first to show an interest, and she was a model in both her sensitivity and her approach. She turned up with none of the trappings of celebrity and a simple request: she wanted to hear from the women themselves about how she could help them.

She arrived at a particularly difficult time. Fighting was raging all over the province. If I'd known then that we would have another decade and more of destruction, I'm not sure I would have found the force to continue. I felt permanently exhausted, the result of working fourteen-hour days all week and often spending a whole night waiting for sleep that wouldn't come. At the time, we were taking in about a dozen raped women a day.

Wamuzila had also returned. The intervening years since her departure had not been happy ones, as she had predicted to my eternal regret.

She came back to Panzi in a coma. She had done her best to rebuild a life for herself in her village. She had started making and selling soap, which provided her with an income and status. She had found a new role in the community, changing how her peers viewed her and other survivors of sexual violence. She once sent me some of her soap with a handwritten note asking me to use it when I washed my hands before surgery.

But her village had been attacked and overrun again by the FDLR, the Rwandan Hutu militia. She had been captured a second time and had gone through similar horrors to the first.

Her attackers had caused another fistula. And she was suffering from meningitis when she was found by Congolese soldiers who overran the rebel camp during a counterinsurgency operation. She was brought to a military hospital in Bukavu, then transferred to us for a second time.

We stabilized her again. She regained consciousness and we began the process of running the battery of tests for sexually transmitted diseases. There was a sickening discovery: this time she was HIV positive. At the time, roughly one in twenty female patients were admitted with the infection.[3]

Once she was strong enough, I scheduled a consultation with Wamuzila in my room. I had to break the news to her about her infection. When I did, she grew angry. She knew that the result was a death sentence. This was before widely available and affordable antivirals offered sufferers a future. She reminded me that she hadn't wanted to leave.

"You made me!" she shouted. "You made me go back all alone!"

Her eyes flashed with anger. She told me everything she thought about how the hospital and I had let her down. She felt she'd been abandoned. She ended by dissolving into tears.

I listened, absorbing her rage, trusting that at some point she would understand that I had done my best for her, that the hospital was always in demand, that there were constant queues of women waiting for a free bed and treatment. I seemed powerful to her, yet I felt hollow and inadequate inside. When she had calmed down, I put my arm around her.

After this second admission, Wamuzila stayed with us for several years. Once she had recovered from the meningitis that may have been linked to her HIV, she needed a whole series of interventions again to repair her fistula. She was still with us when V came to visit in 2007, and she took part in the most important moment of V's trip.

V had wanted to meet as many patients as possible, and several dozen had agreed to share their experiences. They gathered in a hangar at the bottom of the hospital complex. At the time, it was the place where the women ate together.

They sat on wooden benches in groups, dressed in their finest *pagnes* and eager to meet our VIP visitor from New York City. Wamuzila was among them, as were other strong and inspiring former patients from this era, such as Alphonsine and Jeanne.

V went around the room speaking to the women in small groups, helped by a friend of mine, Christine Deschryver, who had overcome her natural suspicion of overseas celebrities and agreed to act as V's guide and translator.

It hadn't been easy convincing Christine to take part. Born to a Belgian plantation-owner father and a Congolese mother, she had worked first as a teacher and then as an aid worker in eastern Congo. After witnessing so much suffering, she had grown cynical about whether Westerners cared about Congo's conflicts and whether any famous visitor would be prepared to show the real commitment needed to make a difference. When I first told her about this extraordinary woman I had met in New York who made vaginas talk, she looked at me as if I had gone mad.

But there was instant chemistry between her and V. They hit it off from day one.

With Christine's help, V asked the survivors to talk to her about their lives. She also shared her own story of abuse, how her father had sexually abused her for years as a child, how she had fled and lived on the streets of New York City, taking drugs and suffering even more abuse. She ended her presentation with a simple appeal: "Tell me what I can do for you."

In return, her audience opened up. V was devastated by what she heard, overwhelmed by the loss and pain. She said afterward that it was worse than anything she had encountered on her travels in Bosnia, Afghanistan, or Haiti.

For her Congolese counterparts, it was a moment of communion and consciousness. They realized that rape occurred not only in the villages and jungles of Congo but in the homes and on the streets of one of the richest cities in the world. A famous, wealthy author from New York was describing the same experiences and emotions they felt.

The atmosphere grew heavy. There were tears throughout, long hugs, and occasional hollow laughs as some of the women sought respite from the heartbreak in humor. V had wanted to hear from the women, and they poured their hearts out.

At some point it became suffocating for everyone. Esther, one of our nurses, suggested some music and a game of follow-the-leader, a technique she uses to shake off the physical lethargy and sense of desolation that can set in toward the end of long group therapy sessions.

Some of the women had brought *ngomas,* the traditional wooden drums played in Congo. They struck up a rhythm. There is something mesmerizing and special about Congolese drumming. The interplay of the beats with the voices and singing produces an effect that sends tingles through my chest and spine.

Everyone was suddenly on their feet, swaying, clapping, and singing, letting the light of the music in. Some of the women formed a line and danced around the hangar, holding on to each other at the waist, rocking from side to side, moving hands and feet in unison. V joined in.

I have always been a reluctant dancer. I rarely take part, even at weddings. But I, too, was carried away in the atmosphere. The women formed groups, taking turns in demonstrating the different dances from the villages and tribes around the region. It felt as if all the pent-up energy and sadness was transformed into joy and happiness in a profoundly spiritual moment.

We danced in the hangar, we danced out the door, and we danced up the slope past the other hospital buildings and toward the main entrance. I did my best to follow in my white doctor's coat, smiling and laughing before the quizzical looks of visitors and other patients.

That night I went home and slept. I slept the whole night, unbroken and untroubled, for the first time in months.

To the question of what she could do for them, V received answers that were almost unanimous. "Every time we think about seeing soldiers again, we're scared," Wamuzila told her. "Find us somewhere we can heal emotionally and prepare ourselves for new lives," Jeanne added. They wanted a shelter, the sort of place that Wamuzila might have gone to after her first operations at Panzi when she had fought to stay with us.

V left telling them she had heard. "I'll do what I can," she said. And she kept her promise.

She approached the head of UNICEF, the UN children's emergency fund, explaining that many of the women who needed help were only teenagers who had had little or no education. UNICEF eventually pledged $1 million in funding.

V launched a worldwide campaign with her V-Day movement focused on Congo. She paid for me to come to the United States to do my first speaking tour at community centers and colleges around the country. For two years, she organized gala dinners and approached wealthy donors in New York and other cities. With her own money, she bought two plots of marshy land from local farmers about a mile from the hospital in Bukavu.

But as the project was finally progressing from the drawing board to reality, she was diagnosed with uterine cancer, which has extremely low survival rates. More than ever, we would need to rely on the work of Christine, who had agreed to become the local director of the project. Her enormous qualities—of single-mindedness, tenacity, and kindness—were vital.

Working together as a trio, we helped turn the vision of the survivors at the hospital into the City of Joy, a safe space for raped women that offers protection, education, and inspiration for its residents. Its motto, written on the entrance wall for all newcomers to read, is "Turning pain into power."

We included Wamuzila, Jeanne, Alphonsine, and women like them from the start of the process: they held meetings with the architect about how to design the spaces. The process was led by them.

So often aid projects fall short when they fail to take into account the people they are trying to help. This sounds so obvious, but you'd be amazed how many times I've seen top-down initiatives designed from faraway offices in Western capitals fail when they encounter the ground realities of Congo.

Once the design work was finished, the construction process began. It was long and fraught with difficulty. For a start, the land was boggy and accessible only via a bumpy mud track that runs past a charcoal market and slums. We faced the familiar problems of electricity and water supply. Finding a reliable builder was a challenge, and the involvement of a UN agency, with its demanding procurement procedures, added a new layer of complexity.

We also insisted that women should be part of the construction team, which would send another message that this was a project not only *for* women but also *by* them. It demonstrated what would become one of our central messages to each future resident: that women are so much more powerful and capable than the positions and roles they are assigned in society.

Female builders were unheard of in Congo, as they are on most construction projects worldwide. The main contractor agreed to take them on with an attitude of utter bafflement, convinced that sooner or later he would have the satisfaction of telling us that women were indeed ill-suited to building walls or doing carpentry.

We identified potential workers at the hospital, some of whom were skeptical and needed vigorous encouragement to sign up to do "men's work." But on site, they turned out to be eager learners and excellent, committed builders.

At the end, some of their male colleagues confessed that the women had inspired them and pushed them to improve and work harder. "This is the story of men and women in the workplace through history," V joked afterward.

She was undergoing chemotherapy in New York as the building emerged from the ground. She'd have regular phone conversations with Christine about the work. Christine would lie that it was going well in order to save V from disappointment. V would pretend she wasn't in pain and hide her constant fear that she would die before the project was completed. All along, the desire to see the center come to fruition helped keep her going. She writes movingly about the process in her book *In the Body of the World*.

When we inaugurated the City of Joy in February 2011, V was there in the crowd of three thousand people. There were also American politicians, aid workers, and a smattering of celebrities, but mostly women from Congo. The women builders were there, too, and they provided one of the most touching moments of the ceremony.

They brought along concrete bricks, which they held above their heads as they danced at the end. They told everyone that they were the first graduates of the project even before it had opened its doors. V organized a grant of $20,000 so they could start their own business.

The idea of the City of Joy was simple: to build on the strength and resilience evident in the women at the hospital. We wanted to do more than help the women come to terms with their traumatic past and face the future with confidence. We wanted them to become agents of change, with the power to make a difference. Once they left, each graduate would serve as an educator and activist, changing perceptions of what a survivor of sexual violence looked like and was capable of achieving.

Every six months, the City of Joy admits ninety new residents. Sometimes they are women from the hospital, other times they are identified elsewhere around the province. Over the years, we've helped train and support a network of health-care providers across the region of South Kivu. They are community workers who assist with fighting disease, improving sanitation, and helping mothers with births. They act as our eyes and ears, often discovering women who have rape injuries and have been forced out of their communities.

Each newcomer to the City of Joy enters through high black security gates that are guarded by former graduates who have been trained for the task. Once inside the campus, they are assigned places in shared stone bungalows set among lawns and flower beds.

They move around on stone walkways shaded by banks of flowering bougainvillea, palm trees, and orange trees. There is a steady tinkle of running water from the streams that run through the site, a reminder of how the area was once marshy and unsuited for construction. Fresh food—pineapples, passion fruit, spinach, and much more—arrives each day from an organic farm that V's V-Day organization has developed, again staffed by former City of Joy graduates.

Presided over by "Mama Christine," the shelter is an oasis of calm, a retreat, a place of harmony that makes the war outside feel like a distant memory. We aim to heal minds and restore bodies. Many of the women arrive malnourished; they all leave stronger and healthier.

Once at the shelter, each survivor follows a series of courses. I teach a segment on gender and female anatomy. I often start by asking how many of those present feel proud to be a woman. A small minority raise their arms. On average, around 80 percent say they would have preferred to be born male. "If I was a man, I could have protected myself," they tell me.

A lot of them identify their suffering as originating in their vagina. It is associated with everything that has gone wrong. "It's because of *that* that I was raped," they say. Their vaginas are the problem, not their attackers or the attitudes of those around them. It also explains their lack of opportunities in life, as well as their sense of rejection.

I encourage them to learn about and accept their physiology. Part of this process is looking at their vaginas. We hand out mirrors so they can do this in private. Many women are initially unable to even say the word for "vagina" in Swahili, *kuma,* and have never seen their own genitals.

Afterward, we draw pictures of the female reproductive system and talk about the different parts and functions. We discuss the menstrual cycle, sex, birth control, pregnancy, and breastfeeding. The first step in learning to love and feel pride in one's own body is knowing and understanding it.

We explain the importance of breaking taboos and speaking openly about female anatomy and sexuality, how the silence around these issues creates the environment in which rapes happen. We stress how shame and embarrassment should always be for the perpetrator, never the victim.

There are also group therapy sessions of between four and ten women, in which they are encouraged to share their personal stories with each other. This is part of the process of accepting and dealing with the past. Sharing helps build trust among the women and makes them realize that no one has to suffer alone.

In separate sessions, they are taught about their legal and political rights. In others, they learn the basics of self-defense, business skills, and arithmetic and literacy for the undereducated. There are sports and yoga. They are also given a choice of vocational training courses: candle or soap making, embroidery, leather working, or farming.

The raucous graduation ceremonies every six months are a life-affirming confirmation of what can be achieved with love. Broken spirits have been turned into militants and powerful women who head back to their villages, not with the stomach-churning fear of Wamuzila but with a desire to change their lives, reintegrate, and transform their communities. I no longer have to wave goodbye to sobbing patients like Wamuzila, who left the hospital the first time unprepared and ill-equipped for her new life.

We don't perform miracles. Not everyone succeeds. With surgery, I can restore and repair the body. The human mind is far more complicated. Each survivor must learn to live with her past, and some wounds are too deep to ever heal completely. Many must learn to live with triggers that revive their traumatic memories.

But every six months another ninety women graduate, extending a network bound together by shared experience that grows stronger with each new addition. A small number stay on to help with the ever-extending operations of the City of Joy, becoming teachers or workers themselves, but most go back home determined to make a difference.

We've observed that many of them become activists for women's rights in their communities or take on other roles as organizers at their local markets or in civil society associations. Having spent a lifetime being undervalued, they spend six months at the City of Joy discovering their own powers and capabilities. And if each survivor helps change the attitudes of just a few people around her, we will achieve what we are hoping for.

Around the same time we opened the City of Joy, we added another institution inspired by the same ideas, Maison Dorcas, which is run by the Panzi Foundation and its tireless and inspirational head, Dr. Christine Amisi. Maison Dorcas serves as a shelter for women with children who are born from rape, as well as for women with incurable fistulas.

The programs are adapted for their needs, but the process is the same: turning pain into power. Hundreds of women have graduated after months of therapy, vocational training, and education.

All of our graduates are then encouraged to take part in and lead mutual solidarity organizations (MUSOs), microfinance initiatives that enable groups of up to twenty-five women to make small monthly contributions to shared savings schemes. Some of the funds are used for small loans to start businesses, while others act as mutual funds for health care, providing a safety net for members for the first time. There are more than two hundred of them around the province of South Kivu, and some have saved up to $3,000.

They are a formidable tool for the reintegration of survivors. The MUSOs are open to everyone but administered by survivors, who often have requests from other members of their community to join once they hear about the benefits.

All of this, sadly, came too late for Wamuzila. Though she was one of the inspirations for the project, someone who made me realize the limitations of a purely medical approach to caring for victims of sexual violence, she was not around when the doors finally opened.

Four years elapsed between the conception of the City of Joy in 2007 and its inauguration. Wamuzila left the hospital for the second time after V's visit and headed back to her village again. I learned later with great sadness that she had succumbed to AIDS.

I take solace only in how her life, marked by so much pain, has helped to alleviate the suffering of others. Her legacy lives on in other women like Jeanne, who was with her during the first encounter with V at the hospital. Jeanne has become one of the most valued staff members at the City of Joy.

In her late teens, she was captured twice by rebels, who subjected her to months of abuse. Like Wamuzila, she was released only after falling pregnant and miscarrying in the jungle. She was eventually rescued but was so weak and sick that she had to be carried to the hospital in a basket, unconscious, the remains of her fetus rotting inside her.

Two other women who were delivered to us on the same humanitarian flight died. We feared that Jeanne would never recover.

She has no family, no children, and will face physical complications as a result of her injuries for the rest of her life. Yet she is living proof that there can be life, happiness, and love even after so much wretchedness.

She shares her story with each new intake of women: the rapes, the filth and stench of her injuries, the multiple rounds of operations. But she tells them that each morning when she wakes up to see the sun rise, she thanks God that she's alive. Her candor, her smile, and her contagious laughter inspire others to open up and reflect on their own experiences.

Now in her early thirties, she's educating herself and working toward her high school diploma. She will dedicate the rest of her life to helping others at the City of Joy and being a voice for the silent sufferers of abuse. Her contemporary, Alphonsine, who arrived at Panzi as an illiterate fifteen-year-old patient, is now a nurse in our operating theaters.

Wamuzila's legacy also lives on in women such as Tatiana Mukanire, who was orphaned as a young child, then raped in Bukavu in 2004 when the town was overrun by forces loyal to sinister Rwanda-backed warlords Jules Mutebusi and Laurent Nkunda.

Their troops went house to house looting, assaulting, and torturing men, women, and children, including several foreign humanitarian workers. We treated around sixteen hundred raped women during and after the three-week siege by their forces.

Tatiana suffered the consequences of her abuse in private, including an unwanted pregnancy that she terminated—despite the law in Congo criminalizing abortion. Her extended family, who had taken her in as a child when her parents died, urged her to keep quiet. She felt she needed to share her story and told her fiancé. He abandoned her.

Despite all of this, she went on to win a place at the university, educate herself, and secure a high-paying job, all while battling alcoholism, eating disorders, and suicidal thoughts. It took her ten years to seek medical and psychological help. When she came to see me, I treated her. She opened up for the first time about what had happened. I could see that beyond the pain lay a woman of extraordinary force.

Today, she has rebuilt her life. She has vanquished her demons. She can never forget her past—she still cries sometimes under the shower in the morning—but it no longer defines or paralyzes her. She became head of a MUSO and is one of the leading members of a new international network of survivors of sexual violence called SEMA that we set up in June 2017. She has spoken at the UN in New York and travels widely to share her experience and inspire other women with similar experiences.

Back in Bukavu, she lives with her husband, a childhood sweetheart, who accepts her and encourages her in her work. When she first raised her plans to become a spokeswoman for other victims, she was nervous about how he would react. "If it's in your heart,

I'll support you," he told her. They've adopted several orphaned children who have become the family Tatiana always dreamed of.

It's *my* dream to see women like Tatiana. She's back on her feet, starting a new life fighting for others. She is demanding that survivors like her are heard and treated fairly. She is loved and loves others, serving as a light for me and everyone she meets.

In 2017, she published an open letter to her rapist. It was an important moment for her, a public admission of her past, her struggles and shame. But it showed how far she had come. "I want you to know that now more than ever, I'm no longer scared of you," she wrote. "You gave me the courage to combat you."

5

IN HIS WORDS

Why do men rape? It's a question I am asked frequently, and sadly it has no simple answer. When I first discovered the crisis in eastern Congo at the end of the 1990s, I was unable to comprehend what I was seeing. It seemed to be the work of madmen and was beyond my understanding as a father, a man, and a citizen. Making sense of it fell outside my competencies as a doctor.

I imagined the perpetrators simply as monsters, overcome by evil, devoid of humanity. My work was caring for the victims; I didn't have the capacity to try to understand their torturers.

Perhaps that was part of my own way of coping, but there are limits to this sort of thinking. Dismissing people as "evil" or "mad," whether they are rapists, murderers, or terrorists, might provide short-term comfort. Dehumanizing them as monsters made me think they were not like me or my peers. But they are, at least they were at some point until they tumbled into darkness and violence.

The war on women's bodies in Congo has not been perpetrated by armies of psychopaths roaming the forests and acting out their sick sexual fantasies. Severe mental illnesses do exist, of course, and can sometimes provide explanations in individual cases. But the rapes should be understood as deliberate, conscious choices and a consequence of the disregard for the lives of women generally, which is the ultimate root cause.

Only by understanding how and why this violence occurs can we try to mount a response at the individual and collective levels—and this holds true for Congo as much as it does for any peaceful country.

I first came face-to-face with one of the men whose violent choices were the cause of so much of the suffering at my hospital on the walkways between the wards and consulting rooms. He was a young man in his early twenties. In his bearing and clothes, he seemed poor and troubled, as if he were carrying a great weight of guilt or shame. Barely able to look me in the eye, he asked if he could see me privately.

I'm often approached by people as I move around the hospital, which was designed deliberately to be open and welcoming. Doctors and nurses mingle with patients and visitors as they walk through the grounds. Depending on my instincts at the time, I usually point people who ask for help in the direction of a staff member and suggest they make an appointment. In some cases, I invite them to come to see me personally in my office.

In our brief exchange, I wasn't sure exactly what this young man wanted. He wasn't seeking medical attention for himself; he wasn't asking for advice or help on behalf of his wife or sister, either. He wanted to talk to me, he said. He had problems and nowhere to go, he insisted. I suspected he wanted money. I told him I was in a hurry and couldn't help.

A few days later, he returned and again approached me with the same appeal. I explained how my time was organized: the demands of my work, the packed schedule organized daily between meetings, consultations, and surgery. I explained, politely but firmly, that I wasn't able to respond to individual demands like this.

On the third time of encountering him inside the hospital, I relented. I figured there must be something urgent for him to keep up his pursuit. His bloodshot eyes looked desperate. I told him he could come to see me at the end of the day once my appointments were finished.

He arrived on time and was shown to my office at the far end of the hospital complex. "Have a seat, tell me," I said as I opened up. I looked him up and down and watched him lower himself uneasily into the chair.

He was slightly shorter than me, with a strong and athletic build. He was dressed in a T-shirt, jeans, and trainers, with his hair razored short on the sides. He clasped his hands in front of him, with his thick, muscular arms showing beneath his short sleeves. We sat down across from each other.

I like to keep my office simple: plain tiles, white walls with the bottom half painted a beige-tan color that hides marks. I have a few framed pictures on the walls for decoration, a bookcase, and lately a glass cabinet where I store personal items such as certificates and prizes.

There is a desk on the far side of the room, and at the other end, I have a sitting area. There are two small couches and two armchairs, all in dark brown corduroy fabric, arranged around a low glass coffee table. I receive everyone here, in front of a window that lets in a wonderful warm light at the end of the day when the sun goes down. Sadly, I've had to have the bottom half blacked out for security reasons.

This is my private meeting area where I sit and listen to my visitors: colleagues, patients, politicians, pastors, priests, and journalists; sometimes aid officials or Silicon Valley technology executives; the occasional foreign minister or UN figure on a fact-finding mission. It's a succession of people that changes every day.

My visitor began by saying he was from the region of Hombo, about one hundred miles west of Bukavu. It's another isolated and thickly forested area preyed on by a variety of armed groups. The main town lies on the river Hombo and straddles the only road linking Bukavu to the diamond-trading hub of Kisangani to the northwest. It takes seven hours to make the short stretch from Bukavu to Hombo. For twenty-five years, until 2011, the road went no farther after the bridge over the river collapsed.

The young man—he said he was twenty—told me he was an orphan and that he couldn't return home for reasons he didn't make clear. He was now in Bukavu, sleeping in the streets, having joined the ever-growing ranks of displaced people with no money and no prospects.

"Can you help me?" he asked.

He said he wanted money to start a business selling palm oil. With $100, he planned to buy himself three large cans and become another one of Bukavu's thousands of street hawkers who sit all day on the roadside, stooped over upturned barrels displaying their fruit, fish, or household products. Every major thoroughfare is lined in this way nowadays, a sign of the poverty and desperation of the population.

I began to probe further. Why couldn't he return home? And was he really an orphan? It's rare in Congo and elsewhere in Africa to be truly orphaned because of the role extended family typically plays. Children without parents are usually taken in by uncles and aunts, as my father had been.

My questioning led him to tell me his story. A trickle of initial information became a great stream, as if he were unburdening himself.

He had grown up with his siblings and parents in a small farming village, he said. They were poor but lived in peace despite the presence of various militias in the region. This changed when he was twelve.

One of the Congolese "self-defense" groups called Katuku attacked. He remembered the shouting and firing, the chaos. Some of the fighters came to his house and marched him away. They pointed their guns at him and told him he had to join.

He was led away into the forest and initiated into the group. He remembers the commander telling him he would be paid and promising him money that never materialized. "You'll also have women. As many as you want," the commander said. He recalled the power he felt when he was given a gun for the first time. He liked the feeling.

Before long, he was taking part in raids at night on villages in the area to look for food, medical supplies, and anything that could be sold to sustain the militia. When they went on operations, the commander would tell his men, "The women are yours, do what you like." The other fighters would capture and rape them. He was only an early adolescent, but he joined in under pressure from the others. It became part of life in the group.

I could feel my hair stand on end. I felt a knot of regret in my stomach for having invited him in the first place. I stared down at the floor and my coffee table. When I did glance up, I could see his haggard features and the dark marks under his eyes. I could see him fidgeting as he searched for his words. Sometimes he'd look up at the ceiling or out of the window into the distance.

I leaned forward in my chair, my hands crossed in front of me. I contemplated standing up and throwing him out. It was disgusting, outrageous, absurd. It was 2014 and I had spent the last decade and a half treating the injuries and devastation caused by killers like him. Of all the places he could have gone to seek help, why had he come to my hospital and sought me out?

But I didn't throw him out. I felt a hot pool of anger rise from my stomach to my chest, then fall away. I resolved to let him carry on talking. He would help me to understand.

He had become addicted to the life of a rebel, he explained. The nocturnal attacks, the gunfire, the action, the killing, the screams. Life in the camp was difficult and uncomfortable, so he found himself looking forward to the operations.

"It was like a drug, I didn't even ask myself any questions," he said. "I actually enjoyed doing bad things."

The reflex of enjoying this sort of action is a condition known as "appetitive aggression"—a lust for violence, in other words— which has been documented in soldiers and security forces all over the world. It was highlighted in a 2013 study by researchers who interviewed more than two hundred demobilized combatants in Congo from sixteen different armed groups.[1]

A majority—64 percent—had started as child soldiers, and more than half said they had been forced to join. A significant number were the victims of sexual abuse from their own commanders.

Many of their statements are bloodcurdling as they describe decapitating civilians, being ordered to beat defecting comrades to death, or consuming human blood or flesh. More than four in ten agreed "a bit" or "strongly" that it could be satisfying to harm others, while one in three felt a "bodily craving or physical need to go out and fight."

My visitor and his fellow rebels had even terrorized people in his home village. They'd returned to kill and rape. They'd taken women hostages who had recognized him as a boy from the area. "How can you do this to us? We knew your parents," they'd pleaded. He smoked drugs and didn't think about it.

But now his past was coming back to haunt him, he said. He had difficulty sleeping and was experiencing regular nightmares. And he had nowhere to go.

"I can't go back to face them," he said. "That's why I want to stay in Bukavu."

I listened, frowning, still mostly staring down at my feet. I wondered whether I could believe what I was hearing. It could just be part of his routine to garner sympathy—and encourage me to part with some money. I wanted to test him.

"What about your parents?" I asked, looking up. "What happened?"

He paused, stiffening slightly, as if a faint ripple of pain ran through his spine. His eyes darted around the room.

"That's the worst bit," he said. "My initiation."

Commanders of armed groups have a variety of methods for breaking in recruits. Many of their new charges are children, who are either abducted or handed over by their parents under the threat of violence. The process is generally the same: brutalizing them, beating them down, then building them back up and demanding loyalty. Discipline is enforced ruthlessly through beatings and murder.

The use of brainwashed children as combatants has been a major feature of the violence in eastern Congo since 1996. As many as ten thousand are estimated to have taken part alongside troops from Rwanda, Uganda, and Burundi during the First Congo War.[2]

Congolese children were lured by the familiar promises of money, guns, and women, then taken to boot camps run by Rwandan army officers. They were "hazed" ruthlessly and exposed to extreme violence, sometimes being forced to execute prisoners in front of their comrades.[3]

During the invasion of Congo, one commander in the Congolese army described looking through his binoculars at the advancing forces and seeing a wave of uniformed kids, some carrying grenade launchers bigger than their own bodies.[4] The head of the rebel force, Laurent-Désiré Kabila, became so attached to his child soldiers, known as *kadogos* (meaning "little ones"), that he made them his personal bodyguards once he was installed as president. One of them was allegedly responsible for his assassination in January 2001.

Since then, the recruitment of children has been a well-documented and widespread tactic deployed by almost all rebel groups in eastern Congo, including the ones backed by Uganda and Rwanda. As well as abducting and forcibly recruiting, they seek out new charges in the ever-increasing pool of destitute children found in cities. The homeless and orphaned are willing to swap their lives of humiliation and poverty for a few hundred francs a month and a gun.

Drugged, brainwashed, and kept in line by the threat of violence and torture, tens of thousands of men and boys with stories similar to my visitor's have taken part in the killing of the last twenty years.

As he began to tell me about his initiation, I felt sure for the first time that he was being sincere. He seemed to experience a traumatic flashback and broke down in front of me. Through tears, he confessed that he had been forced to mutilate his own mother. His commander had sent him back and ordered him to do it as a test of his commitment.

"I didn't have any choice," he said, sobbing. "They said they'd kill me if I didn't. . . . I was only a boy. What should I have done?"

Once he'd finished describing the agony, we sat in stony silence for a few minutes. His breathing was fast and shallow. I could feel my heart beating and the tension in my back and legs.

"She didn't die from what I did to her, though," he murmured finally. "She survived, I know she did. But she died a few years ago, from illness. I never got to go back to see her."

The story of this young man provides a glimpse of what has happened in Congo over the last twenty-five years: the widespread use of child soldiers is part of the answer for why such extreme, sadistic behavior has proliferated. But where did it all start? Why were we suddenly overwhelmed at Panzi Hospital with so many severely injured women in the late 1990s?

The only plausible explanation is that the brutalizing, numbing violence of the Rwandan genocide skipped the border into Congo like a virus once the fighting between Tutsi and Hutu shifted to my country with the two invasions of 1996 and 1998.

From the start of our work at Panzi, we began collecting basic data from patients about the identity of their attackers. More than 90 percent in the early years described their rapists as being armed and speaking Kinyarwanda, the language of Rwanda.

All the horrors seen in eastern Congo occurred a few years earlier in Rwanda during the Hutu-led genocide against the Tutsi: the genital mutilations, the sexual slavery, the rapes in public and in front of family members, relatives forced to abuse and sometimes kill other relatives. It was all documented. Sexual violence was a deliberate tactic used as part of the ethnic cleansing.

Rape was used in Rwanda as a weapon of war, and it is important to understand the distinction between this deliberate and premeditated sort of sexual abuse from the type that occurs in all conflict zones. Rape is an ugly part of warfare just as much as destruction and killing, although it is often treated as a taboo. In every war, soldiers abuse their power by seizing women. These are acts of the conqueror aimed at the "bodies of the defeated enemy's women," as the American feminist writer Susan Brownmiller put it.

The widespread abuse of French and Belgian women by advancing German soldiers during World War II would fall into this category, as would the treatment of German women by soldiers of the Red Army at the end of the conflict. An estimated 95,000 to 130,000 rape victims were treated at the two main hospitals in Berlin alone once the Nazi regime had been defeated, and historians estimate the total number of victims was likely to be in the millions across the country.[5] Abuses by American and British forces have also been documented.

The mass rape of Chinese women by imperial Japanese troops in 1937 in the Chinese city of Nanking saw similarly angry, frustrated, or bored soldiers take revenge for their losses on the civilian population. Approximately twenty thousand cases of rape occurred within the city during the first month of their occupation.[6] In scenes every bit as brutal as anything seen in the forests of Congo, women had bamboo sticks and bayonets inserted in their vaginas and were frequently killed for any resistance.

In Japan, many Allied troops lived up to their nicknames—local women sometimes referred to them as "barbarians"—owing to their sex crimes during the Allied occupation of that country at the end of World War II. And accounts from the Vietnam War include descriptions of gang rape, torture, and genital mutilations by US servicemen that are as sickening as anything you will read in these pages about events in my country.

Rape as a weapon of war is different. It is adopted as a military tactic. It is planned. Women are deliberately targeted as a means of terrorizing an enemy population. Its adoption in conflicts in Asia, Africa, and Europe during the twentieth century can be explained by the fact that it is cheap, easy to organize, and, sadly, horribly effective.

At around the same time mass rapes were being documented in Africa in the 1990s—in Rwanda but also Liberia and Sierra Leone—soldiers in Europe driven by ethnic and religious hatred were adopting similar methods that were just as cruel. During the wars in the former Yugoslavia, Serbian troops and militias deliberately targeted Muslim Bosniak women, even setting up rape camps such as the notorious Partizan Sports Hall in the Bosnian town of Foca.

Rape put fear into everyone, men and women, as much as the threat of death. When the rapes were committed in public, or with the whole family watching, they had a terrorizing effect.

This helped hasten the exodus of non-Serb communities in Bosnia. And by targeting mothers or young victims, the perpetrators damaged the social fabric of their enemies because women were the primary caregivers for their children and the bearers of future generations. By committing the rapes in public, families were destroyed: relationships disintegrated; men divorced their wives out of shame.

Some of the survivors of the wars in the former Yugoslavia later testified in court that their attackers saw rape as a means of permanently undermining their victims' ethnic identity in a way that murder could not. "You should be happy, now you'll carry a Serb baby," some rapists would taunt.

The Rwanda and Yugoslavia conflicts in the last decade of the twentieth century helped raise awareness more than any others about the use of rape for the purposes of ethnic cleansing, leading to important developments in international law, which I will discuss later.

Mass rapes with similar motivations have been observed more recently, in ethnic and religious conflicts from South Sudan to Myanmar to Iraq. In each case, men use it as a means of dominating and destroying "enemy" populations.

Sometimes rape is also used as a weapon in conflicts that have underlying economic motives. It is a way to exercise control over local populations rather than displacing them. In South America, drug gangs use sexual violence deliberately as a means of punishing individuals or communities that threaten their businesses.

The grim particularity of the Congo conflict is that rape has been committed for all of these reasons: by foreign occupying soldiers looking for thrills or revenge, as a means of controlling and cleansing local populations, and for economic reasons.

The Rwandans responsible for the first wave of violence against women were the Hutu extremists who fled into Congo after the genocide in 1994. They were followed by the Tutsi-led Rwandan army and Congolese rebels who took part in the invasions and occupation of Congo in the First and Second Congo Wars in 1996 and

1998. These latter forces showed complete contempt for the rules of
warfare and human rights, committing a string of atrocities as they
moved across the country.

The Hutu who remained after the First Congo War when more
than a million Rwandan refugees returned home formed the vicious
and brutal FDLR militia. They used rape as a way of terrorizing the
local population in areas under their control.

All sides—these Hutu rebels, the Rwandan army, and their
proxies—spread the virus of extremely violent rape much more
widely inside Congo.

By the end of the 1990s, ten different countries were involved in
the Second Congo War, and most of them sent troops. The eastern
part of the country was under the control of the RCD rebel movement, which was backed by Rwanda. The rebels soon splintered
into different factions, however.

Congolese self-defense groups took up arms and sprouted like
mushrooms. Historical land disputes between ethnic groups and
tribes turned violent as law and order broke down. Soon, the whole
of eastern Congo was ablaze. The country was a patchwork of different wars.

What all the different groups had in common was that they adopted the same tactics as the Rwandan extremists and troops. They
caught the virus. They had no regard for civilians. They raped in
public with extreme brutality; they abducted women and led them
into the forests as sex slaves.

Although abuses by the Congolese army were documented in
the 1990s, the contagion reached the national armed forces in a
significant way from 2003 onward. This was the year a peace
agreement intended to unify the rebel-held north and east and
the government-controlled west came into force. It was signed by
Laurent-Désiré Kabila's son Joseph, who had taken power when his
father was assassinated in 2001. All the foreign belligerents were
meant to withdraw their troops and the main rebel militias would
be integrated into the national army.

This policy of absorbing rebels into the national armed forces is known as *mixage et brassage* and has been a constant feature of peace efforts in Congo. Because the government is unable to defeat militias on the ground, it tries to buy them off by inviting them to become regular soldiers, giving them uniforms, and asking them to take an oath to protect the nation. As a result, warlords and thousands of former child soldiers are enrolled in the Congolese military.

This was the case for my visitor. He had decided to come to Bukavu when his commander opted to join the Congolese army. Other abject war criminals continue to serve in the Congolese military high ranks.

Many warlords have been through the revolving door between the military and rebel forces several times. One of them is Laurent Nkunda, whose forces laid waste to Bukavu in 2004, raping thousands of women, including Tatiana, whom I introduced in the last chapter.

Incorporating rebel forces had a major impact on the discipline, cohesion, and effectiveness of the Congolese army. The new recruits laid down their arms and took a pledge to defend the country and its citizens—but they brought their brutal methods with them. Their old weapons were decommissioned, but not their attitudes. We began to document more and more victims who had been abused by Congolese armed forces.

The final jump of the virus, having infected the armed forces, was into the civilian population. Not all rebels were absorbed by the army. Some of them, like my visitor, refused the life of low pay and poor living conditions offered by the military. Instead, they attempted to return to normal life. They looked for jobs. They went back to their home villages if they could. But they kept preying on women. They continued raping.

This vast chain of infection has occurred because the conflict has dragged on for so long. The number of victims, the millions of dead, raped, or displaced, is so shockingly high because the fighting has never stopped, despite the 2002 peace agreement. Eastern Congo is still riven with armed groups nearly twenty-five years after the First Congo War.

And the fuel that sustains the fighting today and explains why rape continues to be used as a weapon of war in Congo lies underfoot. Although the wars had their roots in the Tutsi-Hutu conflict in Rwanda, the fighting is best understood now as having economic, rather than ethnic, causes. It is linked to the mineral treasures that were formed over millions of years beneath the Congolese soil.

Their origins are thought to date back to the Precambrian period, before life even formed on earth. Geologists believe a superheated liquid current rich in metallic alloys surged upward from the earth's core, eventually emerging in the crust of central Africa. As a result, Congo has some of the world's richest deposits of copper, coltan, cobalt, cassiterite, uranium, stannite, and lithium, as well as diamonds and gold. Some are coveted for their beauty, others are vital for our modern technology-based economy.

From the very start of the invasions in 1996 and 1998, our neighbors Rwanda and Uganda set about seizing and repatriating stockpiles of anything of value they found along the way as they advanced through Congo: timber, coffee, livestock, and, of course, gold, diamonds, and minerals.

During the First Congo War, while I was working on the refugee crisis, I remember flying back to Nairobi and stopping in transit briefly in Kigali, the capital of Rwanda. During a wait at the airport, I began chatting with some of the ground crew, sharing what I had seen and what was happening on the ground in Congo. They told me about the unusual arrivals they'd been witnessing: planes laden with crates of gray dust. They had no idea what it was. It was most likely cassiterite, cobalt, or coltan—metallic ores prized by the electronics industry.

A few years later, I attended a dinner party where a local businessman in the mineral trade told us how he had gone bankrupt and lost his life's earnings after the invasion when his warehouse of cassiterite was looted and shipped to Rwanda.

During the first years of the Second Congo War, thousands of tons of minerals and precious metals were flown out of the country, according to a UN investigation published in 2001.[7] Banks and companies headquartered in Uganda and Rwanda handled the pillaging of Congolese resources in areas that were occupied.

The invasion in the late 1990s coincided with a spike in the prices of minerals used by the electronics industry as demand for mobile phones, batteries, and game consoles boomed. The occupation became "self-financing," in the infamous words of Paul Kagame, then vice president and de facto leader of Rwanda. The looting financed the cost of the deployment.

When the foreign countries with troops in Congo began withdrawing their forces from 2002, this threatened the lucrative war economy of mining, logging, and smuggling that had sprung up. The generals and politicians had to find a way of retaining their financial interests. The solution was funding proxy rebel groups. Rwanda, for example, has backed Tutsi militias such as the National Congress for the Defense of the People or the M23 Movement.

These militias always have lofty aims—such as protecting ethnic Tutsi from discrimination in Congo—and adopt absurd self-aggrandizing names that invoke democracy or defense. But they are driven by base economic motives: their business is mining, smuggling, and extortion.

The Congolese self-defense militias also found that running and taxing mines was a means of sustaining themselves and, for a few higher-ups, becoming rich and influential. The majority of these rebel groups have links to Congolese politicians in Kinshasa or to senior Congolese military figures. They are used as muscle to protect private mining interests. For a politician, control over a militia means leverage, giving him influence and the ability to bring peace or wreak mayhem.

The weak Congolese state collaborates with these actors. It has been unable to take back control of its territory and regulate the industry because of a deliberate policy of neglect and underfunding of the armed forces and the state bureaucracy. I always say that the chaos in eastern Congo is an organized chaos. It serves the interest of a network of figures that stretches to the upper levels of the Congolese state as well as to the elites in our neighboring countries.

Rape is part of this process of ruthless exploitation. The twenty-five years of sexual violence in Congo is bound up with the plundering of raw materials.

First, the supposed availability of sex became part of the recruitment process for militias, as my visitor explained, an enticement along with guns and power offered to new recruits. The same tactics were adopted in Iraq and Syria by the ideologues of the Islamic State (also known as ISIS), which set up an elaborate system of sexual slavery. Young men and boys are told they will have as many women as they want. Rape is part of the initiation process and a sick bonding exercise among recruits.

But sexual violence is also part of the military strategy of commanders. Rapes are carried out as a way of disciplining anyone suspected of failing to support the rebels. If a community is suspected of being hostile—by working with the Congolese armed forces or a rival militia—the women are targeted.

It also serves as a method of dispersing civilian populations around mining areas. Once minerals are discovered at a new location, there is a rush there among artisanal miners that often leads to conflicts over ownership and control of the land and water. Mass rape is used to evict the local population. It's not ethnic cleansing, as in Rwanda or the former Yugoslavia. It is rape used as a weapon of war to clear an area for personal enrichment.

In 2009, we conducted the first research of its kind that looked into whether there was an explicit link between incidences of extreme sexual violence and the known locations of major mineral deposits. Our hypothesis was that the abuses were concentrated in areas where there were mining operations.

The research paper, which I authored jointly with academic Cathy Nangini and published in the *PLOS Medicine* journal, used data on the origins of the victims we were treating at Panzi. We found that three-quarters of them came from three isolated rural areas—Walungu, Kabare, and Shabunda—where rich deposits and mining operations under the control of armed groups were known to exist.

The map we produced, overlaying areas of high rates of rape and reserves, was a striking visualization of how sexual violence was linked to the struggle for control of minerals, precious metals, and diamonds.

So who ultimately benefits from this chaos? The warlords, of course, who are near the top of the pyramid. They accrue the taxes and are often involved directly, or through associates, with the trading of these conflict minerals. They use the income to pay their men and buy new weapons.

Above the warlords sit the members of the business, political, and military elite—they are usually overlapping categories—who live in mansions and drive expensive cars in the Congolese, Rwandan, and Ugandan capitals. They orchestrate the smuggling, then the first stages of processing, and finally the exports to markets in the Middle East and Asia. They work with a host of shady businessmen and multinationals, who help launder this bloodstained production, injecting it into global supply chains.

Minerals such as coltan, cobalt, tantalum, and tin remain essential raw materials for the electronic products that sustain our modern economies and lifestyles: for the capacitors, circuit boards, and batteries found in everything from mobile phones to electric cars to space and satellite technology. Congo is the world's biggest producer of cobalt, used in rechargeable batteries, and has the world's largest known reserves.

Rwanda in particular has become a leading world exporter of minerals in quantities far beyond its own reserves and production capacities. Along with Uganda, it is also a leading supplier of gold, which has been a cornerstone of the war economy for twenty years. Almost all of Congo's gold production is smuggled out, and this pattern continues now just as strongly.

In a June 2019 report, UN experts on Congolese raw materials found that Rwanda declared exports of the metal to the United Arab Emirates (UAE), a leading global gold-trading hub, of 2.16 tons. But UAE statistics showed imports from Rwanda to be six times that level, at 12.5 tons. Uganda declared exports of 12 tons, but UAE data showed imports of 21 tons.[8]

This is why in my Nobel Peace Prize acceptance speech in Oslo in 2018, I challenged the assembled audience of dignitaries and anyone watching on television to examine their own consciences. Slick consumer-brand marketing is intended to make you forget the dirty secrets of the production process. Congo's mines, where men and boys put their lives and health at risk hacking away in unlit tunnels or at vast open-cast sites, are the filthiest, most obscure, most overlooked end of our modern global economy.

"When you drive your electric car, when you use your smart-phone or admire your jewelry, take a minute to reflect on the human cost of manufacturing these objects," I said in my Nobel speech. "Turning a blind eye to this tragedy is being complicit." I wasn't ac-cusing anyone, but I wanted to make sure everyone listening knew they could no longer ignore the reality.

There has been some progress to clamp down on the theft and laundering of Congo's raw materials. The Organisation for Economic Co-operation and Development has developed guidance for compa-nies using tin, tantalum, tungsten, and gold from Congo, requiring them to check on their suppliers.

In 2010, the United States passed the Dodd-Frank Act, which includes a section requiring US-listed companies using minerals from Congo or the region to perform due diligence and report on their supply chains. Twelve African countries, including Congo and Rwanda, also have legislation in place requiring companies to check their supply chains.

These measures have had an impact in some areas, but the incen-tives are so huge, the markup on smuggled minerals and precious metals so great, that corrupt criminal networks still find ways to profit. From the port in Bukavu, boats leave regularly at night, slid-ing over the silent waters of Lake Kivu toward unloading spots in Rwanda where border guards look the other way.

Sadly for Congo, the plundering of its natural resources for the gain of a narrow elite is a pattern repeated throughout the history of the last two centuries. It has taken different forms, at first benefiting European colonialists, then Africans. But the methods and objectives are always the same.

The first traders who exploited the territory with no regard for its inhabitants came in the eighteenth century: the Portuguese sailors and Arab traders who ventured down the coasts of Africa looking for slaves.

Then came rule by Belgian king Leopold II, who set the borders of the modern country with his Congo Free State. His criminal, extractive regime focused initially on ivory. The elephant herds of the equatorial forests were decimated and their tusks shipped to Europe, where they were shaped into the era's luxuries: billiard balls, piano keys, chess pieces, sculptured ornaments, and false teeth. Then came a new boom driven by the invention of the rubber tire in 1888.

The king's administrators, working with locally trained Congolese soldiers, used forced labor and collective punishments to drive the locals into the forests to tap wild rubber trees. The shocking greed was matched by extreme brutality. If production quotas were not met, whole villages would be torched, women would be taken as hostages, and thousands of people had their limbs cut off.

The tyranny of his rule, immortalized in photographs of men, women, and children with severed hands or feet, is estimated to have cut Congo's population in half. Mass murder, disease, starvation, and exhaustion all took a toll. The birth rate plummeted. Millions of Congolese lives were lost. Adam Hochschild, the American author of the best-selling book *King Leopold's Ghost*, concludes that the killing was "of genocidal proportions."[9]

Belgium took over the Congo Free State in 1908 amid international outrage over Leopold's misrule, which had sparked the world's first international human rights campaign, orchestrated from the United Kingdom and vigorously supported by Mark Twain in the United States. Tributes and statues of Leopold still abound in Brussels alongside the grand public works of his era financed by

Congolese labor. Only now, thanks to the Black Lives Matter movement, has a reckoning with this past forced its way into the present.

Belgian rule from 1908 coincided with a boom in the price of metals as Europe militarized. Congolese copper was soon in high demand for artillery shells during World War I. Congolese uranium was later used in the atomic bomb dropped on the Japanese city of Hiroshima at the end of World War II.

The country's mineral riches explain why it was inconceivable that independent Congo in 1960 could depart from the West's orbit. When Prime Minister Patrice Lumumba began looking to the Soviet Union for support, this was the signal for Belgium and the United States to begin plotting his assassination.

Mobutu's four decades in power afterward merely continued the exploitation of Congo's mineral wealth for narrow personal gain. Instead of Europeans, he and his network of cronies grew tremendously wealthy as the country grew poorer.

Over the last twenty years, revenues from Congo's minerals could have been used to develop public services—the schools, roads, hospitals, and armed forces that I and my fellow citizens so desperately need. Instead the money has been siphoned off, mostly into private pockets but also into the public accounts of our neighbors, who enjoy the jobs, tax revenues, and foreign exchange earnings brought from selling smuggled Congolese resources.

China, which has secured vast mining rights for itself over the last decade through opaque deals with the government of former president Joseph Kabila, is the latest overseas power to spy opportunities for self-enrichment. The pattern of exploitation continues.

Even when tax is paid to the Congolese state from foreign investors, barely anything reaches the people because of the endemic corruption that Kabila did nothing to tackle over his eighteen years in power. The campaign group Global Witness estimated that $750 million of mining revenues paid by companies to state bodies was lost to the treasury in just two years between 2013 and 2015, representing a fraction of the total.

This is the story of Congo, one of the richest countries in the world that has been laid low by 150 years of foreign occupation, dictatorship, and ruthless exploitation.

The young man who came to my office in 2014 was just one tiny piece of this vast, complex picture. His life had changed the moment the local Mai-Mai militia attacked his village. He didn't say who gave the commander his orders or whose interests the militia ultimately served. He had no idea who pulled the strings above him.

After listening to him for nearly an hour, I had heard as much as I could bear. I felt strongly that I wanted him to leave. By way of bringing the conversation to a close, I told him that he was a young man and that he had his life before him. He should try to make amends for his sins and find new meaning.

There is a charity in Bukavu called BVES that works with former child soldiers, providing them with support, counseling, and training. I scribbled down the name and number and recommended that he contact them. And out of a mixture of pity and a desire to hurry his departure, I said I would give him the $100 he was looking for.

As he got up to leave, I found myself asking a last question, almost involuntarily, as we stood facing each other. For so many years, I'd tried to visualize the sort of human being who could inflict such wanton damage on a woman's body. Now I had one before me.

"But why did you need to rape with such violence?" I said. "I've never been able to understand. You can't imagine the things I've seen here over the years. Why mutilate someone?"

His reply chilled my blood.

"You know, you don't ask yourself any questions when you slit a goat's neck or a chicken's. A woman is like that. We did what we wanted to them," he said.

He left. I closed the door behind him and slumped back down into my armchair, playing over in my mind what I'd heard and trying to make sense of it. I pinched the bridge of my nose and rubbed my eyes. I shook my head in disbelief.

Throughout his descriptions, his halting, sometimes jumbled sentences, I didn't sense he had come to me to seek forgiveness or even that he felt remorse for the lives he'd taken and the others he'd spoiled. He seemed to feel a tug of guilt over his mother, but that was all.

He was bound up in self-pity and sorrow for his own miserable condition. He wanted help for himself, not advice on how he could atone for his past. But to my surprise, as I sat thinking over the conversation, I felt a sense of pity for him, too.

Shorn of his gun and sense of power, he was a pathetic sight, weak and damaged. He was clearly suffering from post-traumatic stress disorder and, without help, faced a spiral of more nightmares and misery.

How should I feel toward him? He was at once a perpetrator and a victim of violence, a child brainwashed and misled who was turned into a killer. The real guilty parties were the adults who had consciously and knowingly manipulated him. They were the cowards ultimately responsible for his actions.

He was like so many Congolese who have been sucked into the conflict and then spit out. We are all traumatized survivors in one way or another, each with our own painful experience of loss, counted not just in missing loved ones but in lives derailed and dashed ambitions.

I kept thinking about his parting statement. It was so cold, so casual, so matter-of-fact. Raping women had bothered him no more than killing a goat or chicken. He never worried about the pain he inflicted because it sated his own sexual and violent de-sires, like cooked chicken or goat satisfied his hunger. That he would speak about women in the same breath as animals made clear how little importance he attached to their lives. It showed a horrifying lack of respect.

As I contemplated his behavior in the days afterward, I realized that this truly wretched individual had something in common with all rapists. He was an extreme example, for sure, but his attitude was similar to the suited businessman who forces himself on an underling, the drunk student who attacks a contemporary, the respectable family man who rapes his wife, or the Hollywood producer who bullies actresses into bed. Because whenever a man rapes, in any situation, in any country, his actions betray the same beliefs: that his needs and desires are paramount and that women are inferior beings that can be used and abused.

Men rape because they do not hold women's lives to be as valuable as their own. And when they feel they can use their power for their own sexual gratification and get away with it, they take advantage.

A breakdown in law and order in a peaceful country can give a glimpse of what happens when men feel they can get away with abusing their power. In such circumstances, sexual violence tends to surge. There is now a body of research into the vulnerability of women at such times and how emergency responses need to be "gendered" to take into account their specific need for protection. New Orleans provided a telling example in 2005 after Hurricane Katrina.

There was confusion about the extent of sexual violence during the lawless aftermath of the storm that flooded the city. At the time, there were some exaggerated media reports of mass rapes that were subsequently discredited. But two academics from Loyola University found widespread evidence of an increase in sexual crime in research published in 2007.[10]

Much of it resembles wartime crime: a popular jazz singer recounted being woken up and assaulted at knifepoint as she slept on her roof. Others were snatched while doing shopping or grabbed while returning to their homes. Reports of "stranger rape"—in which the victim did not know the perpetrator—leapt. In peacetime, they are a small minority of the total cases.

The largest number of reported assaults—31 percent—occurred at shelters or evacuation sites, such as the city's Superdome, according to a survey by the National Sexual Violence Resource Center in 2006. That survey found evidence of forty-seven assaults—the tip of the iceberg given the difficulties in locating victims and their reluctance to come forward.

The way women are treated during wars and natural disasters should be seen as an explicit manifestation of the violence inflicted on them behind closed doors during peacetime. Sexual violence is a global epidemic that we are only just starting to tackle.

The figures vary according to countries. In a major survey in the United States, commissioned by the Centers for Disease Control and Prevention, one in five women (21.3 percent) reported that they had suffered rape or attempted rape at some point in their lives.[11] That's roughly twenty-six million women. The figures suggested that 1.5 million women suffered rape or attempted rape every twelve months. Over their lives, 43.6 percent experienced some form of sexual violence.

In the United Kingdom, the number of women who reported rape or attempted rape since the age of sixteen was significantly lower at 3.4 percent, in a study published in 2017. But 20 percent said they had experienced some type of sexual assault, such as un-wanted touching or indecent exposure.[12] The figures are roughly the same for Australia.[13] In France, one in seven adult women (14.5 percent) said they had experienced sexual violence at least once during their lives.[14]

In a landmark report in 2018, the UN Office on Drugs and Crime called the home "the most dangerous place for women." The pri-vate sphere is where the overwhelming majority of abuse of women and girls takes place, not in the forests of Congo or the ISIS slave markets.

Worldwide, almost one-third (30 percent) of all women who have been in a relationship have experienced physical and/or sexual vi-olence by their intimate partner, according to a 2013 World Health Organization study.[15]

When sexual violence occurs without consequences for the per-petrator, it becomes tolerated. And once a practice is tolerated, it ends up forming part of the culture. Rape with extreme violence in Congo spread and became anchored in the population because it became normalized as a way of treating women. But sexual violence is also normalized in almost all societies and particularly inside some institutions, such as the military, universities, prisons, or even Hollywood.

Every two years, the US Defense Department publishes the results of a study on sexual assault in the armed forces based on a survey of one hundred thousand members.[16] The initiative is to be applauded. It demonstrates that progress is being made in acknowledging the problem.

The US military is far more transparent and systematic than its equivalents in other countries in trying to root out sexual violence. It has spent hundreds of millions of dollars trying to sensitize recruits in the last ten years. But the latest figures are astounding, giving us an idea of the incidence of rape in other armies around the world and the scale of the challenge in stamping it out.

In its 2018 survey, it found that one out of every sixteen military women reported being groped, raped, or otherwise sexually assaulted *within the last year.* Only a third of cases were reported to superiors. In the US Marine Corps, one in ten surveyed women reported being assaulted, twice the rate of the army and the air force. The youngest and lowest-ranking women were found to be most vulnerable, with most perpetrators found to be peers rather than more experienced and senior officers.

University campuses are another place where shockingly high levels of sexual abuse can be found. Surveys show that on average in the United States, between one in five and one in four undergraduates experience some form of unwanted sexual contact.

A study released in 2015 by the Association of American Universities surveyed 150,000 students at twenty-seven colleges and universities, one of the largest of its kind. It found that 27.2 percent of female college seniors reported some unwanted sexual contact—from being molested to penetration—which was carried out either by force or while they were incapacitated because of alcohol or drugs. Around half of the victims reported forced penetration or attempted forced penetration.[17]

The rates were even higher in Ivy League institutions. At Yale University, 34.6 percent reported being assaulted, 34.3 percent at the University of Michigan, and 29.2 percent at Harvard University. The surveys found that queer, gay, lesbian, or transgender people faced the highest levels of abuse of all.

Universities and the military, along with prisons, are institutions where high levels of documented sexual violence have spurred media attention, investigations, and action to change the culture of gender relations and sexual behavior. But all organizations, from businesses to associations and parliaments, have a responsibility to take action. If they are not combating sexual violence, then they are tacitly tolerating it.

The battle therefore must be led in changing how women are viewed by men, elevating them from second-class citizens, from objects or property, to equals. And it must be backed up by measures that place a cost on committing a crime, whether it be in a war-torn country like Congo, a disaster zone, a university campus, or a bedroom. I will expand on my ideas for leading this combat in the coming chapters.

I never again saw the former child soldier who came to my office in 2014. I don't know if he used my money wisely, whether he started his business selling oil and created a new future for himself. I don't know if he sought help for his psychological problems. I doubt it. He never went to see the organization I recommended to him.

In case you were wondering whether I should have informed the police after his confessions, I can assure you that there would have been no point. There are thousands of demobilized former fighters like him roaming the streets of Bukavu. Our barely paid security forces have neither the resources nor the motivation to investigate their crimes.

Other than a few organizations like BVES that try to help them, they are left to their own devices. One recent aid program handed out motorbikes to demobilized fighters so they could earn a living by carrying passengers. The result was an increase in aggressive behavior on the roads as these young men sought a fleeting adrenaline fix by driving their vehicles at reckless speeds.

The former combatants are part of the legacy of our decades of violence. Even if the fighting stopped today, their untreated psychological problems will be with us for generations.

He made me reflect on how his life might have turned out differently. There was nothing inevitable about the choices he made. Why was he so unabashed, so lacking in remorse for his actions, unlike my patients, who were burdened by the stigma and shame associated with his crimes? How might his destructive impulses have been stopped, along with the men who were instrumentalizing him? Had he been educated differently as a boy, might he have resisted the lure of guns and the rape culture of his militia in the first place? I turned those questions over in my mind endlessly. And the answers are relevant not just for Congo but for the rest of the world.

6

SPEAKING OUT

The first and most important step in combating sexual violence is speaking out about it. I want to tell you about a twelve-year-old girl who made me think differently about my own role. The year was 2006, just over three years after a peace deal that was supposed to put an end to the war in Congo but proved as ineffective as we feared at the time. That year 1,851 survivors sought help for their injuries at our specialized rape clinic. Most had been attacked in their homes at night. More than half had been gang-raped.[1]

It was a time when I would often return home punch-drunk from a day of racing between consultations and surgery, worried about our finances and filled with despair about the endless stream of patients.

We were vastly improved in how we helped them, physically and psychologically, but we were still years away from the holistic treatment program we offer now that includes more specialized care as well as reintegration programs and vocational training. The City of Joy and V's help came later.

We had started efforts to go outside the hospital to try to tackle the root causes of the rape crisis, not simply the consequences we saw every day with each new admission. Part of those efforts saw us start an outreach scheme with the local military courts. We would meet army magistrates who presided over court-martial proceedings against Congolese soldiers accused of rape. We had noted the sharp rise in cases involving former rebels who had been integrated as regular soldiers in uniform as part of the *mixage et brassage* policy.

Only a small number of aggressors faced a court-martial, and they were always the low-ranked ones, not commanders or the top brass. But we saw the meetings with military judicial officials as an opportunity to explain our work. Our documentation and medical reports were often used during proceedings and our doctors would sometimes be called as witnesses. But our work was still widely misunderstood.

In March of that year, we had a high-ranking visitor who was the chief medical examiner at the military court in the capital, Kinshasa. After arriving in his jeep, the general was shown to my office, where I greeted him at the entrance.

I was immediately struck by his size. His giant silhouette filled the door frame. He must have been well over six feet tall. His thick arms stretched the material of his uniform as he stuck out a hand to shake mine firmly. Polished medals dangled at his lapel.

We sat down and I thanked him first for the interest he was showing in our work. I delivered a brief presentation of the hospital and an explanation of how the women admitted in Panzi were only the tip of the iceberg, the most severe cases of a problem that was widespread across eastern Congo. He nodded and listened.

I mentioned our work with the military courts and outlined how we prepared our medical reports. We had trained staff to take forensic notes and photos of the injuries they saw when necessary. In their reports, they would include testimony from victims that was sometimes presented as evidence in court. They made assessments as doctors on whether the wounds were consistent with an assault.

I mentioned the unfortunate case of one of our doctors who had been jailed recently by a magistrate after she failed to appear as an expert witness during a hearing. She had sent a note in advance to say she was handling a medical emergency, but the magistrate had taken no notice. We had to pay bail to free her.

He nodded some more. He sat with a look of polite attention, listening but with an expression that indicated I should not take too much of his time. I suggested we take a walk and invited him, if he felt it would be useful, to meet some of the patients. He agreed.

He moved through the hospital with the confident step of a senior military figure. He passed in front of the turned heads and stares of patients and their families without acknowledging them. Most Congolese are instinctively nervous around men in uniform.

We arrived at the wing reserved for survivors of sexual violence. It has its own wards and public areas for the women and girls, as well as dedicated operating rooms. Around fifty women had gathered in the space where they socialize, a large open-sided hangar. They sat at long wooden tables, curious yet apprehensive about meeting our visitor.

As we began, I explained who he was and why he was at Panzi, and then I invited any of the women present to ask questions or recount their own experience if they thought it would be helpful. Several of them seized the opportunity.

Our visitor stood with feet apart and arms crossed, listening respectfully, his face a picture of firmness. Several women took turns to give brief accounts of their assaults, each one harrowing and painful in their individual ways. Then a young girl stood up to talk.

I hadn't met her before, but she gave her name as Witula and her age as twelve. She said she was from the region of Shabunda, the resource-rich enclave from where a constant stream of victims limped out to the hospital. She was slightly built, with hair cut short.

"I was out in the fields with my mother when suddenly there was shooting everywhere," she began. She spoke clearly, with the pitch and innocence of a child, and also the directness. Her confidence was impressive for someone so young. She paused and took a breath. She composed herself for a second or two, then continued in a voice that gathered strength the more she spoke.

"People began running in all directions. I tried to follow my mother. She was running back towards the village. It was all very confusing," she said.

"I was behind my mother but not running as fast as her. Suddenly I felt some hands around my waist and I fell down. The next second I was on the ground and I felt a big weight on me, a man. I couldn't move. He was much heavier than me," she said.

She described how other rebels ran over—they were from the FDLR, the extremist Hutu militia from Rwanda. Their machine guns were slung across their backs. She was dragged from the field where she had fallen toward some bushes.

She screamed, she said, so hard she felt her lungs were going to burst. People were still running in all directions. She could hear more gunfire and other cries. No one heard her. Or if they did hear her, no one came to help.

"I had never been with a man before," she said. "I screamed and screamed. It hurt so much. I asked them to take pity on me, I begged them."

The room had fallen completely silent.

I was standing next to the general, and as she spoke, I saw his look of confidence and self-assurance suddenly falter. It was as if a small crack had opened up on a brick wall. As I glanced across, I could see him tensing the muscles of his jaw. Perspiration was gathering on his forehead. His eyes became watery. "How could anyone do this to a girl like that?" I heard him mutter, shaking his head in small movements. "How is it possible?"

Witula continued. As she spoke, some of the women stared at the floor, while others had tears in their eyes as they looked at the girl with sympathy and admiration, imploring her to go on.

She didn't know how many had raped her. The last of them had stabbed her in the genitals. She said it was a knife, but it could have been a bayonet, whose injuries I had seen dozens of times.

"I don't remember what happened next. I just lay there. I thought I would die and I begged God to end the suffering and pain. But once the firing had stopped, people dared to come back to the village. They found me in the field, covered in blood. I had passed out by then. They brought me here," she continued.

At this point, there were tears visible on the general's cheeks.

Some of the other women had started crying, too. As the girl neared the end of her story, each wretched new detail rang out in the silent room. There was just the low background hum of the generators working nearby.

The general could bear no more. He began to sob. Everyone's gaze turned from the girl to him. Then his knees buckled.

He fainted, falling hard onto his back.

It all happened so quickly that I was unable to react. There wasn't time to grab him under the arms. Shrieks rang out. The calm turned to commotion.

I rushed forward and helped put him in the recovery position. A colleague ran to get an oxygen mask. The women crowded around him, dozens of anxious faces, frozen with fear, looking down on his prone figure. Some of them began fanning him.

After a couple of minutes, he regained consciousness. We helped him back to his feet and he walked unsteadily to one of the doctors' rooms nearby. We checked his pulse and put him on a drip. We asked whether he had a medical condition that might explain his reaction.

"No," he assured us. "It was hard, very hard," he said. "I had no idea anyone could treat a child like that."

Once he felt strong enough, I accompanied him back to his jeep, where his driver was waiting. He looked sheepish. He thanked me for the presentation and for our work as he closed the door.

I have no full explanation for why he reacted the way he did. As a military man he should have been aware of the atrocities committed in our region. Had he chosen to simply close his eyes and believe the government and army propaganda, that the reports were exaggerated or made up by people with an agenda against the country?

Did it revive his own traumatic memory, recollections of events that he had suppressed? Did he think of his own children while listening to the girl? Perhaps he felt an overwhelming sense of failure, of the military institution he served, which failed to provide security. Or perhaps something larger, how we had failed collectively as adults to provide protection for our children.

I can only speculate. But the experience, one of the most unforgettable visits I've ever had, was an important milestone in my personal journey. It meant the work we were doing with the military justice system was having an impact. I felt sure this man would be changed by the experience, that he would be more willing to believe the victim, to view medical reports as vital evidence.

It was also validation of the work we were doing to help rebuild our patients' confidence and encourage them to speak out and press charges. In the supportive environment of the hospital, Witula had managed to give full expression to her suffering. She and other women from Shabunda, who were always the most outspoken, served as an inspiration to others who were struggling to overcome their feelings of shame.

Above all, I and everyone else in the room had witnessed a demonstration of the power of words. It was like David confronting Goliath. Witula had ignored her status as a poor "victim" from a remote farming village and felled this towering figure with the strength of her testimony. She felt no shame—why should she?—because society had not yet infected her with the lousy notion of "honor."

I felt as though I had witnessed a particular form of the power of women that I have encountered in other situations since. Women have an ability to cut through the brittle exteriors of men, who pride themselves on projecting force and invulnerability. These macho masks are designed to be intimidating, but they can be pierced. They are no match for real inner strength.

The experience with the general made me question if I should change how I saw myself. I still considered myself first and foremost a physician. My place had always been in a white coat or in surgical scrubs. I spent almost all my time at the hospital. But the speech by this fearless girl was an inspiration. It seemed like a call to do more.

I had been doing my best to alert others about the crisis whenever there was an opportunity. I made myself available to journalists whenever they made inquiries in Bukavu. I briefed UN agencies locally about the situation on the ground. I had helped researchers from Human Rights Watch when they prepared the first major international report on the issue of extreme sexual violence in Congo in 2002, entitled *The War Within the War*. We also compiled detailed but anonymized data on patients and their injuries, which we saw as an important public service.

But I concluded that I needed to work not just as a doctor but as an ambassador for my patients, to use my position as head of the hospital to carry their stories as far as possible. In the same year the general fainted, 2006, I was given an opportunity to do so thanks to another influential visitor.

Jan Egeland, who at that time was UN under-secretary-general for humanitarian affairs, organized a trip to eastern Congo and requested some help to prepare his meetings. He was the highest-ranking official at the UN to express an interest in our work at the time.

We helped organize a series of events for him, both in villages that were badly affected by violence and at the hospital, where he held private sessions with survivors. After our experience with the general, we thought it safer to offer one-on-one chats or meetings with small groups. It was a considerable amount of work, which we embraced as a rare opportunity to spread awareness. Hundreds of women came forward offering to speak to Jan, seeing him as an intermediary with access to powerful people who might bring an end to the country's suffering.

Toward the end of his trip, I remember him coming to my office for a meeting that deeply affected him. It was with a woman who told him that she had gone into the forest to look for firewood to prepare dinner for her family. Her husband and children were waiting for her, she said, but she didn't come back. That is the painfully familiar beginning of so many of these stories.

She was snatched and taken away by a group of around thirty rebels of Rwandan origin. They took her to a camp and tied her to two trees, a rope on each outstretched limb. The ropes were so tight, they ended up cutting the blood supply and severing the nerves in her hands and feet.

When she did eventually make it back to find her husband and children, she had to be carried. She could no longer walk. She told Jan about her experience from her wheelchair.

I could see the impact. Jan and I had already spent a considerable amount of time together, and I had grown to like him for his energy, commitment, and compassion. After the woman left and we were alone again, he seemed troubled. As he sat on the brown sofa in my seating area, he slumped down.

He puffed his cheeks and let out a sigh. He closed his eyes momentarily and rubbed his jaw with his hand. He had temporarily lost his natural sparkle, a great quality that was evident when he arrived in Congo.

"Thirty days like this," he said disbelievingly, spreading his arms and legs. "I just can't . . . I mean, how is this still happening?"

I've seen many people react like him over the years, stuck for words to express their disgust, incomprehension, and anger. This is our daily reality in eastern Congo.

The resilience of the survivors at Panzi Hospital, the passion with which they spoke to him, and their desire for the world to bring an end to the fighting left a permanent mark on Jan. He mentioned the meeting with the woman in the wheelchair at a press conference when he returned to New York.

He was so touched by what he'd heard and so outraged that Congo's women were not an international priority that he suggested I travel to New York to address the United Nations.

Receiving his invitation was like a thunderclap that startles you. It felt like one of those moments of acceleration in life, when events lurch forward at an uncomfortable pace. If anyone had told me at the beginning of that year that I'd be addressing the UN by the end of it, I would never have believed it.

But a few months later, in September, I flew to New York, knowing that I was being given a platform to speak on behalf of the women who had shared their stories with Jan. It was a task that I accepted with humility and a degree of trepidation. I knew that if I could find words with a fraction of the power of those used by the girl with the general, then perhaps I could make an impression on the governments in attendance and urge them to put an end to the atrocities.

Since the year 2000, the UN had become more active and had been slowly expanding its peacekeeping effort in Congo. Known initially as MONUC, it eventually became the largest force operating with a UN mandate. But generally speaking, the fighting and torture continued under the mostly indifferent gaze of world leaders.

Correspondents working for major international media companies would fly in occasionally for a week's reporting, but there was little appetite for news from a distant war zone with its apparently incomprehensible slaughter. No world power saw its interests threatened in Congo. Rwanda continued to receive strong financial and diplomatic backing from the United States and the United Kingdom in particular. No influential leader considered ending the conflict among their foreign priorities.

I arrived in New York a few days in advance and began my preparations by contacting the Congolese diplomatic mission. I was hoping for some guidance and help. I thought, naively in retrospect, that we were on the same side in looking to find solutions to end the suffering of our country. I'd worked on my speech in Bukavu and had fine-tuned it on the plane on the way over. I planned to submit it to the ambassador first.

That year, the first free presidential elections in Congo in forty-one years had taken place. Against the odds, and with financial support from the European Union in particular, millions cast a vote for the first time in their lives. It was inspiring and moving. The vote resulted in victory for then thirty-five-year-old Joseph Kabila.

He had taken over the reins of power when his father, Laurent-Désiré, was assassinated in 2001. He campaigned mostly on his record as a peacemaker, having signed the 2002 Global and Inclusive Agreement that was meant to bring an end to the fighting. Despite the ongoing violence in the east, where militias and Rwanda continued to fight, the people of South and North Kivu backed him overwhelmingly, seeing him as the best hope for stability and peace.

I was not among his supporters, which put me at odds with many of my peers. I was unconvinced by his peacemaking and troubled by his lack of vision. He seemed to have no real program for tackling the country's other problems: corruption, malnutrition, and lack of infrastructure. I told everyone that I hoped I would be proved wrong, that he would prove a more effective leader now that he held a democratic mandate for the first time.

Despite my personal misgivings, as I arrived in New York, I was ready to support his government in all its efforts to improve the lives of Congolese citizens and end the fighting. I believed we had a common interest in acknowledging the rape crisis and using the resources and influence of the international community to end it. I called the Congolese embassy and asked if I could speak with the ambassador.

First, I was told he was out of town. When I called back, I was offered a meeting, but he never turned up.

The next day, I took a taxi from my hotel to the UN complex building on East Forty-second Street. I was to speak during a session on sexual violence in conflict zones that was being chaired by the UN's secretary-general, Kofi Annan, and attended by Jordanian princess Haya Bint al-Hussein and Jan Egeland.

Shortly before taking our seats, I spoke briefly with Kofi Annan. He asked if I had met the Congolese envoy. "No," I replied. "It hasn't been possible." He looked puzzled.

We walked out into the huge auditorium. I felt a flutter of nerves. I'd done plenty of public speaking before, particularly in churches in Bukavu, but addressing the world's diplomats was a very different proposition. I took a deep breath and patted my suit jacket a final time, checking that a copy of my speech and my glasses were still in the inside pocket.

Each of the UN's 193 member states had been invited. As I settled into my seat on the stage, I looked around at them arranged in a giant semicircle in front of us. Each country had a desk. At the front sat the ambassadors, with their advisers placed in chairs behind.

I looked at the name plaques, checking off countries in my mind: Australia, China, France, Germany, the United States, the United Kingdom . . . Each space for their delegations was filled. They sat impassively, wearing headphones and waiting for our speeches, which would be piped to them in each of the six official languages of the UN.

My eyes darted around the room, seeking to locate the Congolese desk. When I found it, I felt an electroshock of disappointment. The desk was empty. No ambassador, no advisers.

Throughout the whole of my speech, my gaze would return there every time I looked up to glance at the audience, as if drawn to a bright light. It was a dazzling void. The seats remained unoccupied throughout. It suddenly made sense why the ambassador had never returned my call or turned up for our meeting.

I've told you previously about the administrative problems we faced in Bukavu from the beginning of our work at Panzi Hospital: the lack of public funding, the corruption, the attempts at extortion. This was the first time I realized how I was seen by the new government under Kabila: I had been boycotted, but most important, the patients at my hospital had been boycotted. I was in New York acting as their envoy. The empty chair made it clear that speaking on their behalf, drawing attention to the plight of Congolese women, was unwelcome.

To make matters worse, afterward I was approached by the ambassador of Sudan, who objected to my raising the mass rape of women by the government-backed Janjaweed militia in Darfur.

"How can you claim this?" he said indignantly. "Where is your evidence?" I pointed him toward the numerous reports from both the UN and human rights organizations working in the country.

The whole experience was a salutary one in some respects. I mentioned in the introduction how I've often felt as though my personal journey has been one of understanding with ever greater clarity just how difficult it is to be a woman and a survivor of sexual violence.

My treatment at the UN was an education in how women are so often received whenever they find the courage to denounce their attackers. They are told to keep quiet, to avoid causing a scandal or embarrassment. Progress has been made in recent decades in some countries, but the instinct to cover up, ignore, disbelieve, or intimidate people who speak out remains depressingly common and deeply ingrained.

Breaking the silence about sexual violence in all its forms—harassment, rape, incest—is the essential first step in tackling the problem. As I mentioned in chapter 3, many of the first patients at Panzi Hospital would make up improbable stories to try to explain their injuries. They would blame them on an accident. They were oppressed by societal pressure, which encouraged them to suffer in silence or face stigmatization and ridicule in public.

Smashing this taboo is essential for several reasons. First, sexual violence thrives in silence. Keeping quiet creates an environment in which men can continue to abuse with impunity. It serves their interests. For as long as knowledge of a problem is suppressed, the same destructive behavioral patterns are allowed to continue.

Second, self-censorship stops women from drawing strength from each other. In our work in Congo, we place great emphasis on group therapy, in which women are encouraged to share their stories with each other. At the City of Joy, the inspirational Jeanne, whom I told you about in chapter 4, helps with this process.

By sharing, survivors often realize that they are not alone in their suffering, that others also face the same struggle with pain, rejection, and guilt. Role models such as Jeanne are proof that the future can hold promise and possibility.

Third, speaking out serves as an education for all, particularly men. Only then can we begin the process of changing public policies, educating boys differently, and making men understand the consequences of sexual abuse that often leaves such deep psychological wounds.

Let me be clear, too, that I understand and respect the decisions of some women not to share their experience. No one is obliged or put under pressure to take part in group therapy sessions at Panzi. It is not the right approach for everyone. There are a host of reasons that may motivate someone to deal with an assault privately. Nobody should suffer an added layer of torment by feeling guilty for deciding not to denounce her attacker.

But it is true that we can produce the societal and cultural changes that are needed only if we work collectively—this requires people who have not experienced sexual assault to speak out against these atrocities as well. We are all a part of this system, and all play a crucial role in righting it. This is why the #MeToo movement of 2017 was such a watershed moment. I watched it unfold with jubilation from Bukavu, seeing how it galvanized so many women to speak openly for the first time in public.

Campaigners working on sexual violence had been pushing for decades to encourage more open discussion about the prevalence of rape and other forms of abuse. After meeting V in New York in 2006, I had helped support a campaign with her called Breaking the Silence, as well as a UN campaign called Stop Rape Now in 2010 that enlisted celebrities to help bring sexual abuse out of the shadows.

Previous campaigns had all laid the foundations. The Take Back the Night movement in the United States from the 1970s had worked to call out rapes and attacks on women. More modern equivalents include Hollaback!, which was founded in 2005 in New York, and even more recently It's On Us, an initiative started by the Barack Obama–Joe Biden White House in 2014. The 2018 movement Time's Up built on this leadership. A host of national campaigns by feminist organizations around the world each made contributions.

But the #MeToo movement was able to reach so many more women than all previous attempts at taboo smashing. It was supercharged by social media and the fact that celebrities shared intimate stories about their own experiences, rather than just reading scripted messages condemning violence against women.

Never before and with such great numbers had victims of sexual abuse dared to speak out simultaneously. It seemed like a global group therapy session, with each new addition and revelation empowering others to find words to express their own experience. So many men woke up in the process to the sheer pervasiveness of aggressive sexual behavior at companies, in offices, on the streets, and in bedrooms.

Many women did not feel moved to post on social media, but the public outpouring sparked important conversations in private. Wives and girlfriends shared previously undisclosed stories. As V has noted, it did not lead to men issuing apologies and promising to atone for their past bad behavior. But many examined their own consciences.

And yet the old instincts didn't take long to reappear. Tarana Burke, who began the Me Too idea in 2006, wondered publicly if in fact it was a watershed at all. Part of her concern was that ethnic-minority women did not feel represented, as the media coverage focused initially on the revelations from Hollywood actresses against powerful white abusers such as Harvey Weinstein. There was also a major backlash.

I wondered when the counterattack would begin. It didn't take long, and opponents used various spurious arguments. All of them were aimed at returning the subject of sexual abuse to a place where we could pretend not to know about it, like a shameful family secret at a gathering of relatives.

They relied on one of two arguments: either that sexual abuse was being exaggerated and did not merit the attention it was receiving or that the accusation was so serious it should not be raised so brazenly against men who could not defend themselves.

Some critics claimed that all men were being portrayed as predators and wrongly slandered. Women were exaggerating or simply making up stories, said others, repeating a favorite trope that women are prone to making up vindictive stories about sexual assault. Conservatives and some politicians in developing countries dismissed the movement as a sign of the sexual depravity of rich, bourgeois society or the decadent, liberal West.

One of the most notorious counterattacks came from a group of privileged, high-profile women in France, including actress Catherine Deneuve, who claimed #MeToo risked ruining the game of seduction. It implied that sexual harrassment was both an inevitable part of the dating process and, when it did occur, nothing to dwell on. Arguments about protecting women were being used "to lock them in their roles as eternal victims, poor little things at the mercy of phallocratic demons," the women wrote.

The message from all the opponents was the same one broadcast to me by the empty chairs of the Congolese delegation at the UN: that it was better to keep quiet. When victims of sexual violence or campaigners refuse to be quiet, they frequently find themselves subjected to intimidation.

In 2019, I attended a conference in Norway to discuss the problem. There were hundreds of delegates from women's groups, aid agencies, and officials from various countries at a hotel in the capital, Oslo. One of the speakers was a Ukrainian woman, Iryna Dovgan, who had joined our international platform for survivors.

Iryna told the audience about the prevalence of rape and the abuse of women in eastern Ukraine, which has been under the control of separatists backed and armed by Russia since 2014. When she had first spoken in public, she had seemed unsure of herself. In Oslo, she spoke confidently and fluently.

Iryna, then fifty-two, had been detained by separatists in her hometown of Yasinovataya, where she ran a beauty salon. She was falsely accused of being a spy for the Ukrainian forces, which were shelling the area in a bid to wrest back control from the rebels.

During her interrogations, she was beaten, tortured, and threatened with gang rape. She was then tied to lamppost in public for hours, where passersby were invited to insult and assault her. An investigation by the United Nations Human Rights Monitoring Mission in Ukraine in 2017 found significant evidence of sexual abuse in detention centers run by government and rebel forces.

After the end of the session in Oslo, the delegates gathered for a buffet lunch, typically a time of introductions and small talk. Iryna was approached by a man who said he was a Russian diplomat. She found herself standing alone with him as others chatted around her.

"I listened to your speech with interest," he began. "How can we be sure what you say is true?"

Iryna was taken aback. "It's my own story. I lived through it," she replied. "Why would I come here to make up a story?"

"You should remember that we Russians and you Ukrainians are one people," he continued, his voice growing more menacing. "Do you realize the shame you are creating by speaking like this in front of people?" He finished by telling her she should stop defaming Russia.

She came to see me afterward and described what had happened. She was visibly shaken and had experienced the exchange as a clear attempt at intimidation. Attending events like this one and speaking in public required courage. I could see her resolve was being tested.

Iryna continues to attend conferences and speaks about her experiences just as forcefully as ever as she works to raise awareness about the extent of the problems in eastern Ukraine. But had she not had the backing of family and colleagues, including members of our international survivors' network, she might have been tempted to abandon her work.

It is vital for women to receive continued support, not just at the time they decide to break their silence but in the months and years afterward. Intimidation can be far more explicit in other cases, but it always has the same objective: silencing the victim.

Several women abused by Harvey Weinstein testified in court how he would wield his influence and power in the movie industry with the same chilling threat if they suggested they would complain. "You'll never be part of this business," he'd say, or, "You'll never work again."

Media reporting on the Weinstein cases also led to a spotlight being cast on how he and other powerful men and organizations used lawyers to silence their victims when threats and intimidation were judged insufficient. Nondisclosure agreements, or NDAs, which are often imposed as part of a settlement in sexual misconduct cases, prevent a victim from sharing her experience with others—and allow her attacker to keep on abusing with impunity.

In one such case, it was revealed how Olympic gold medalist

gymnast McKayla Maroney was pressured to sign an NDA with USA Gymnastics after complaining about abuse from elite sports doctor Larry Nassar. This culture of covering up allegations of abuse within elite US gymnastics silenced victims and enabled Nassar to carry on abusing. He was arrested and jailed for life only in 2018, after decades of pedophilia. In total, more than 150 victims came forward to testify against him in court.

Since the #MeToo movement erupted, more than a dozen US states have passed legislation limiting or banning employers from forcing their employees to sign NDAs as a condition of employment or as part of a settlement for harassment or sexual abuse. One, New Jersey, has made NDAs unenforceable.[2]

In the most patriarchal societies, intimidation is far more explicit and socially acceptable. So-called honor crimes, in which a raped woman is attacked and sometimes killed by her relatives, are part of the conspiracy to keep women in a state of fear and mute compliance. Rape is viewed in these communities as a source of shame and even as a form of adultery.

In 2000, the United Nations Population Fund estimated that five thousand women and girls were murdered each year in "honor crimes," not just for rape, often for simply attempting to choose their own partners rather than the men selected by their parents. Many more murders are disguised as suicides or accidents, so the statistics, as so often when it comes to violence against women, are likely to be an underestimate.

The overall homicide figures of women globally also tell their own story. Men make up the overwhelming majority of homicide victims worldwide. Most of them are killed by strangers. But women are usually killed by someone close to them.

Global Study on Homicide, a report published in 2019 by the United Nations Office on Drugs and Crime, found that of eighty-seven thousand women intentionally killed, 58 percent had been murdered by an intimate partner or family member. The most dangerous continent for women was Africa, followed by the Americas.[3]

So-called honor crimes and all other forms of domestic violence and intimidation of women have a chilling effect on survivors who want to speak out and denounce their attackers.

The case of a seventeen-year-old girl who was raped in the northern Indian state of Uttar Pradesh in 2017 in what became known as the Unnao scandal is another dispiriting tale of how going public often comes at enormous personal cost.

India has begun to tackle the endemic problems that make the country one of the most dangerous places in the world to be a woman. Mass protests in New Delhi and other cities in 2012 sparked by the gang rape and murder of a twenty-three-year-old physiotherapy student on a bus were a milestone for the country in terms of public acknowledgment of the problem and the difficulties faced by women. But progress has been patchy.

Outside of the relative wealth and privilege of middle-class areas in cities, life remains highly patriarchal, with strong notions of female "honor." The caste system also makes low-status women especially vulnerable. The underperforming and frequently corrupt security and judicial systems make it exceedingly difficult to seek legal recourse.

The Unnao case five years after the New Delhi protests illustrated how much work still needs to be done. In June of that year, the victim, a low-caste girl from a village in India's largest state, Uttar Pradesh, was lured to the local leather-making town of Kanpur. She was told by a neighbor in her village that she would find work. Instead she found herself imprisoned, gang-raped, and trafficked. One of the people who raped her was Kuldeep Singh Sengar, an upper-caste politician from her village who had risen to become a state legislator during his two-decade career.

When she escaped from her captors, she made her way back to her family and did what few women in her position dare to do, because of the fear of retribution or pressure to keep quiet from their families: she filed a police complaint against Sengar.

The 2012 New Delhi rape case had cast a spotlight on how Indian police so often ignored or failed to follow up on sexual assault cases.

Perhaps she believed the claims that the country had changed in the meantime. But the police refused to register her complaint against the politician, and a doctor who examined her recommended that she drop her demands for justice.

Showing extreme bravery and courage, she persisted. When police in her village didn't react, she went over their heads to the local court, then to the regional police, and eventually to other politicians. All the time, her family was being threatened. Local police arrested her father on trumped-up charges. He was so badly beaten up that he died of his injuries in custody.

Several days after her father's arrest, in a state of utter desperation, the girl tried to set herself on fire in front of the office of the state governor. Although police intervened to stop her, the attempted immolation attracted national media attention to her plight. The federal police were brought in to investigate and Sengar was finally questioned and arrested.

But this was not the end of her ordeal or the final price she would pay for defying a powerful man. As she was driving with her lawyer and two aunts several months later, a truck swerved onto their side of the road and hit their vehicle head-on.

Her aunts died. One of them was a key witness in the case. The girl needed intensive care but survived.

When Sengar was finally convicted of rape and handed a full-life sentence at the end of 2019, more than two years after attacking her, the victim had spent years being threatened and called a liar in public. She had lost her father and been badly injured herself. Her actions demonstrated extraordinary power, yet it is likely that the lesson for many other women reading or hearing about her sacrifices is that it would have been better to keep quiet.

This is the way in which silence is maintained. In many parts of the world, women are kept in a constant state of fear. They are told from birth that the essence of their womanhood and their value lies in their "honor," meaning their sexual purity. They know that losing it can be a disastrous source of shame and possibly a death sentence.

Forcing women to think first about their "honor," not their right to a life free of violence, is the most pervasive and powerful tool used to keep women quiet across the world when they are victims of sexual abuse. The threats, beatings, mockery, and sometimes murders of those brave enough to speak up serve to reinforce the rules. Simply put, denouncing sexual violence is dangerous in many parts of the world because it challenges the vested interests of men.

Once I had decided to expand my work to being a mouthpiece for the women of my hospital, not just their doctor, I began to be subjected to various forms of intimidation myself. The snub during my first speech at the UN in 2006 was part of this pattern.

The threats have taken different forms over the years. Sometimes it's a menacing phone call at night or an anonymous text message. The worst ones warn me about dangers to my wife or daughters. I've had people fire off automatic weapons into the air outside my house. Even on the occasion of my mother's funeral in December 2019, I was threatened with an attack during the drive to our native village, Kaziba.

It's impossible to know who is responsible. The threat is constant but also so diffuse that it is very difficult to guard against. Anyone who has an interest in suppressing the truth about the conflict in eastern Congo and keeping women quiet sees me as an adversary.

It's not always people connected to the government. Some of my enemies are individuals accused of rape by women treated at the hospital. We provide free legal services at Panzi to encourage patients to press charges against their attackers. The accused are sometimes powerful men with businesses, political careers, and reputations to protect.

Warlords, politicians, and senior army officers with an interest in sustaining the violence in eastern Congo as cover for their pillaging and smuggling of minerals and precious metals also see my lobbying work highlighting their activities as a threat to their incomes.

And my insistence that justice must one day be served for the estimated five million dead and missing, the war crimes, and the hundreds of thousands of rapes in Congo that have resulted from the First and Second Congo Wars threatens everyone with blood on their hands, including our foreign neighbors Rwanda, Uganda, and Burundi.

There have been several attempts on my life since the attack on my first hospital in Lemera. In 2004, during the occupation of Bukavu by renegade army generals, gunmen sprayed ammunition into my private office in the center of town. A bullet went through my empty office chair. I would have been sitting in it had a friend working for an international humanitarian group not called me and insisted I meet him for a cup of tea just minutes before.

I also owe a debt of gratitude to the United Nations peacekeeping force and senior UN officials, who have arranged for a team of peacekeepers to stand guard outside my house around the clock. Almost continuously since 2013, they have provided protection and accompanied me on my rare trips outside. Without them, I would have been compelled to leave Congo.

Although I live with a constant and nagging feeling of insecurity, I am also aware of my privileges. I can count on several supportive nongovernmental organizations (NGOs), a handful of sympathetic UN officials, and overseas friends. Through my work, I have come to know people in the government and military. The woman in Unnao, India, had none of this. She took on the powerful on her own. Across the world, when women speak out, they often do so unshielded and alone.

The snub at the UN in 2006 made it clear that the new government of Joseph Kabila saw me as an adversary, not as an ally, in the fight for the dignity and safety of our fellow citizens. The message was stated with ever-growing clarity and menace in the following years.

Even after my first speech at the UN, I still spent most of my time in the hospital working as a doctor and surgeon, but I was making a conscious effort to travel and speak more widely. I began to feel more and more disgusted and outraged: with our own government, with our neighbors, with the companies that exploited our misery, with the international community for not acting more forcefully. For each woman we treated, I knew there were thousands of others who would never make it to the hospital.

I felt let down by Western powers—the United States and the United Kingdom continued to shield Rwanda—but also by the African Union, the regional grouping of African states. Its silence and feebleness are a stain on the organization, which resembles a unionized club of leaders who look out for each other's interests. Instead of working to end the slaughter of Africans, they protect each other.

My lobbying work began to bear fruit in terms of personal recognition abroad. In 2008, I won the UN Prize in the Field of Human Rights and the Olof Palme Prize, a Swedish human rights prize, which were both accepted in the name of my patients. The only joy I felt was that their voices were starting to break through.

I also began working on a PhD that year, first at the University of Ghent in Belgium and then at the Université libre de Bruxelles (ULB; Free University of Brussels). My aim was to share what I had learned through bitter experience, hoping it might help prevent suffering somewhere else in the world and raise awareness in medical circles. The subject of my doctoral thesis—the treatment of low-traumatic uro-genital and intestino-genital fistulas—is a sad summary of the skills I have acquired over the years.

In 2011, we had a case that disgusted and outraged me to such an extent that I concluded I was still not doing enough. It was an inflection point, when my transition from being a doctor to a campaigner gathered pace. My mission to speak out about Congo took on new urgency.

A mother and a child around eleven years old came to the hospital. There was something familiar about the mother, I thought. She walked with a limp, probably caused by polio contracted in her childhood. They were from Mwenga, an area southwest of Bukavu.

She confirmed what I feared: she had been treated in Panzi in 2000. She had been among the first waves of patients whom we had treated for rape injuries in the years after we opened. She had been attacked at her home and then abandoned by her husband.

She had come to the hospital needing treatment for her injuries—genital lesions and an infection—but she was also pregnant with the child of one of her attackers. She was extremely traumatized and needed the best we could offer at the time in terms of psychological support.

Like many women in her position, she was terrified about the idea of giving birth to a child who would remind her daily of her suffering. When she delivered her daughter, whom she called Wakubenga (meaning "She who is scorned"), she rejected her and refused to breastfeed.

Many mothers in her position can never accept their child. The daily torment of being reminded of the conception and the wrench of conflicting emotions is just too much to bear. What's more, they know the child will be a drain on their limited resources. What chance do they have of marrying them well or seeing them find a good job in a society that stigmatizes and excludes them?

I've had former patients drop their babies at the door of my office. We have infants abandoned outside the hospital at the security gate on a regular basis. Others arrive in tears, confessing that they had taken their child to the bank of a river and were about to toss them in.

We have a special team nowadays to help mothers and children in these circumstances. Much of the work is done by our extraordinary *mamans chéries,* the nurses turned social workers who accompany each patient. They support the mothers and also work with the families of patients, sometimes undertaking visits in person to resolve tensions with husbands and parents.

We deliver, on average, about 3,000 children at the hospital annually. Some years as many as 15 percent, or around 450, have been children born from rape. Our specialized center, Maison Dorcas, now offers accommodation, care, and psychological support for these new mothers.

With time and the prompting of staff, Wakubenga's mother had been able to see that her child was as innocent as she was, that they were both the victims of their aggressors. By rejecting her, she would only have added to the misery and suffering she felt. It takes extraordinary strength to reach this point: the power to love unconditionally. A majority of women who give birth to children born from rape at Panzi succeed in accepting their children.

But there are many who do not. Some simply walk away, or they accept but then deliberately neglect them as they grow up. The children find themselves shunned by their parents, siblings, and peers, often deprived of education and cursed in public. We had one woman who referred to her child, in his presence, as *interahamwe,* a widely used term for Rwandan extremists.

We have no idea how many children share this fate, but I call them a "ticking time bomb," children born from violence who grow into adults having never known love or affection. There was a survey carried out just in the town of Shabunda in 2008 that concluded three thousand children there had been born from rape out of a population of half a million.

Just over a decade after we had discharged Wakubenga and her mother from Panzi, both of them returned. Wakubenga was now a preteen. And to my horror, I learned that she had been raped, too, and was also pregnant.

It was almost too barbaric and twisted for me to comprehend: a child who had been born from rape had been raped herself and was now expecting a child. The problem was becoming multigenerational.

Later that year, in 2011, I was invited to address another panel on sexual violence at the UN in New York, this time on the sidelines of the General Assembly, the annual gathering of world leaders. I was invited by the Office of the Special Representative of the Secretary-General on Sexual Violence in Conflict, a UN mandate established in 2009 and directed by a brave and dynamic Swede, Margot Wallström. I left for New York with Wakubenga on my mind.

Compared with 2006, this time would be different. Five years earlier, I had gone to seek out the Congolese ambassador, thinking that he might help me. By now I knew that I could expect only obstruction from my own government. It was a surprise, therefore, when a cabinet minister sought me out instead.

Shortly after arriving, I met an old friend of mine who had left Congo years earlier to take up a senior position at the UN in New York. We had a drink together at my hotel in midtown and exchanged news. I told him about Wakubenga and my despair at the passivity of the international community. He left wishing me luck with my presentation.

But later that evening, he called me again. He said he had received a message from the staff of Congo's health minister at the time, an ally of President Kabila's, who wanted to invite him and me for dinner. Was I interested in accepting the invitation?

I was surprised to say the least, but given the strained nature of my relations with the government, I agreed. I figured it might be an opportunity to clear the air, especially with a minister who might be more sympathetic than his cabinet colleagues given his portfolio. I said I'd be happy to accept, and the following evening we were invited to his hotel.

He was staying in the five-star Waldorf Astoria, like many foreign delegations when the General Assembly was in session. The entrance hall was buzzing with people moving in all directions as I arrived. Staff, diplomats, and businessmen rushed in and out through the entrance doors, where liveried staff were ushering people into black limousines waiting outside.

I made my way to a private dining room where we were meant to eat together. I was shown to a table where the minister and my friend were already seated. It was very private: there were just the three of us.

I remember the fairly formulaic pleasantries exchanged at the beginning. I remarked on the impressive activity in the reception area and our very luxurious surroundings. He seemed very familiar with it. I imagined President Kabila upstairs in one of the suites.

Once the waiter had taken our order, he got down to business.

"So, Doctor, what are you doing here in New York?" he asked.

"I'm being given a prize by the Clinton Foundation," I explained. This was the truth, but also an elision. The Clinton Foundation had decided to give me their Global Citizen Award at a ceremony after the General Assembly. I thought it unwise to bring up the UN speech immediately.

"That's good. Is it all? I've heard you are also going to speak at the UN as well, no?" he said, feigning ignorance. "What time is it?"

"I was invited by the special representative to talk about the situation in South Kivu tomorrow," I replied. "I'm planning to—"

I was about to tell him what I intended to say. I wanted to give him the latest admission figures for Panzi, even raise the case of Wakubenga. I assumed he wanted to know what I intended to say, to make sure that I wasn't going to attack his government publicly. He cut me off midsentence.

"The president is going to be making his address tomorrow at the General Assembly. I called you here to give you some advice," he said, pausing and leaning over the table toward me. "If I were you, I wouldn't make your speech."

The words were spoken calmly but with intent. I scanned his face up and down to ensure I had fully understood the message, finding only seriousness and menace.

"If you do it, you know it will be impossible to guarantee your security back home," he continued darkly, gesturing with his hand in the air as if motioning back to our country, thousands of miles away and a different world from our expensively carpeted dining room.

I felt as if something had suddenly got caught in my throat. I felt short of air. Was he really threatening me here, over dinner in a quiet corner of the Waldorf Astoria?

"But Minister, my—my speech has been scheduled," I stammered. "There are several heads of state who have said they plan to be there. We need to raise awareness. This is something we should—"

"Let me be a bit clearer. If you do it, you'll be making a choice, because you won't be able to go back to Congo afterwards. It'll be too dangerous for you," he added. "Do you understand?"

I felt the walls closing in. For days I'd been imagining myself returning to the UN, seeing the diplomats and politicians in front of me with their headphones. I felt emboldened this time, more confident, ready to voice my frustration and anger. I sensed the whole scene being ripped away.

"I understand your concerns," I replied. "But perhaps I could show you my speech beforehand? I could make some changes. I'm sure there's a way we can agree."

I knew I was climbing down, but the only solution was to try to negotiate. He wasn't interested.

It was obvious he had been sent to deliver a message. There didn't seem any possibility of getting through to him. He was impervious to any argument or appeal I might make to his conscience. He spoke to me with the superiority a minister might feel in the company of an uppity small-town doctor from a provincial hospital, which is surely how he viewed me.

The food arrived and a plate dropped softly in front of me. I stared down at my salad, suddenly having no appetite and feeling an overwhelming desire to leave and find a space to think, to work out what I was going to do next.

The rest of the meal passed in a blur. The minister regained his genial affect of the premeal small talk, neither embarrassed by the threat he had just delivered nor bothered by my obvious discomfort. Once he'd finished his main course, his mission accomplished, he made his excuses and left.

I walked back to my hotel with questions running urgently through my head. Should I, could I defy him? It was outrageous to intimidate me like this. But then how could I hope to live and carry on my work back home? What about Madeleine and the children? I would be putting them in danger, too.

I made my choice back at the hotel. This was a warning I had to take seriously. It wasn't a death threat delivered in the middle of the night down the telephone. It was a minister acting like a mafia figure, making no attempt to hide his identity or the intent of his words.

I called Margot Wallström and told her what had happened. I explained that under the circumstances, I would have to cancel. She said she understood my decision and asked me if I felt safe at the hotel. She said she'd inform then secretary-general Ban Ki-moon.

The next day, I had a visit from several US officials from the State Department, who took a statement about what had happened. They asked me if I needed protection, an offer I declined. I explained that I'd canceled my speech and intended to return home.

I stayed in New York to receive the Clinton Foundation award at a ceremony at the Hilton Hotel. Former US president Bill Clinton presented it in a room packed with wealthy donors and a host of American celebrities. I delivered a brief speech explaining our work and urging everyone to wake up to the conflict in Congo. But my mind was elsewhere.

I wanted to get home to see Madeleine. I felt raw and shaken inside. During the day of return travel, as I sat in my airline seat, I played over and over the conversation at the Waldorf Astoria. The journey felt like an eternity.

Threats and intimidation of survivors of sexual violence come in many different forms: from their attackers, from the families of their attackers, from community leaders and public figures, and even from their own families. Those who speak out in spite of all these pressures need our support. They demand our respect. They deserve recognition for the power they demonstrate by refusing to be cowed.

Madeleine was waiting for me when I finally arrived back in Bukavu. I felt guilty for exposing her to danger. Perhaps I had been unwise or overly confident, blinded by my own righteous anger, in wanting to speak out in New York.

She reassured me in her usual calm and wise manner. There would be other opportunities to speak overseas, she said. I had retreated, but only in order to carry on with my work.

There were indeed other opportunities. I bottled up the admiration I felt for the young girl who had made the general faint and the women who had shared their experiences with Jan Egeland. I stored the outrage I felt over the life of Wakubenga.

The next year, I was invited again to the UN. I was asked to join a panel that included the first woman president of Chile, Michelle Bachelet, and then British foreign secretary William Hague. I felt bold enough to accept.

Another assassination attempt followed. I still get flashbacks of the gunfire, the screams in the dark, the crumpled body of a dear friend who sacrificed his life to save mine. Another unsolved crime, another attempt to keep sexual violence in the shadows.

7

FIGHTING FOR JUSTICE

*I*n early 2014, I couldn't take it anymore. Over the previous two years, we had admitted a succession of children with appalling injuries at the hospital, all from the same village, Kavumu, about twenty miles from Bukavu. It began with a few isolated cases, but over the following years we received dozens more.

They had all been seized in similar circumstances. In the dead of night, men broke into their family homes and would often administer a powerful sleeping agent to their victims. Once kidnapped, they were raped, then returned, bloodied and confused, in the morning. Each devastating case represented a childhood wrecked; the extent of the injuries and scarring meant as adults most would never be able to have normal sexual relations or bear children.

In the first five months of 2014, we had fifteen very young girls. The final straw was a four-year-old who was brought to the hospital with severe recto-vaginal injuries. It was disgusting, heartbreaking, and simply beyond my comprehension.

I operated on her with my friend and longtime partner, Guy-Bernard Cadière, the Belgian surgeon who is a specialist in laparoscopy, a type of abdominal keyhole surgery, and treating fistulas. He visits Bukavu regularly with his team from the ULB medical university in Brussels. As well as fundraising for our work and serving as a constant source of advice, he has helped train our surgeons to use his noninvasive techniques.

There are few things that can shock a surgeon. The inside of the body holds no mysteries for us, but we operated on that girl while choking back tears. As we examined the injuries, we wondered aloud how they had been inflicted. We worked by turns in shell-shocked silence and in animated fury.

At the end, I flicked off my gloves, changed into my coat, and walked back to my office, lost in angry contemplation, feeling nauseated and repulsed. How many other girls would they mutilate before being stopped?

Once I had calmed down, I resolved to visit Kavumu in person. I needed to see with my own eyes and hear from the community about what was happening. Why were families unable to protect their children? What were the parents doing when their children were grabbed and abused like this?

I struggled again with a feeling of powerlessness. It felt as if I were always picking up the pieces, stitching back together shattered bodies, traumatizing myself in the process, but without ever being able to envisage an end to the violence. I needed to hear from the mothers and listen to the fathers in person.

Working with several humanitarian groups, we set up a meeting at a local community center a week later. I traveled with my escort of UN peacekeepers. We invited the top prosecutor from Bukavu, who agreed to attend, as did a senior officer from the Congolese armed forces and a representative of the police. The governor of the province and the regional interior minister agreed to attend but backed out at the last minute.

The level of interest could be gauged by the number of people who turned up: there were around five hundred in total, packed into the stifling room. Some sat two to a chair, others stood at the back. There were even people milling about outside for want of space.

The atmosphere was charged from the beginning. There were mostly women in the crowd, many fanning themselves in the thick, warm air. They were speaking loudly among themselves as we took our places, some sending accusatory glances toward the prosecutor and police as they sat down.

Years of pent-up frustration came spilling out once they were given the microphone and invited to talk. They described how the community lived in constant fear. They all went to sleep never knowing if they would wake up and find a child missing or be startled by the sound of armed men bursting open the flimsy doors of their homes in search of a new victim.

Some women's rights activists implored the men present to do more. "Do you have no pity?" one of them told the room. "This is not about rape, it's about the massacre of our children!"

The prosecutor spoke, telling the crowd that his hands were tied unless parents came forward and filed criminal cases. "You need to denounce what is happening," he urged them. "If you don't file a complaint, then it is very difficult for me to do anything." There was a ripple of indignant chattering. Some of the mothers near me rolled their eyes.

Once he'd finished, the prosecutor found himself in their crosshairs. He was mocked as "Monsieur Hundred Dollars" because of his reputation for bribe taking. The culprits were never arrested, a local community organizer said to applause. And if they were, they could buy their freedom.

"They carry on because they can get away with it. They know they won't have any trouble," he explained.

As well as the string of rapes, there had been murders, arson attacks, and beatings around Kavumu. A local activist who had begun investigating the rapes had been gunned down in his home in front of his daughter. In a sign of the widespread insecurity, even an army camp nearby had been attacked.

Several people hinted they knew who was behind this wave of exactions, but no one was willing to name names. "We know if we say anything, we'll be killed, too," said the community organizer. "This night might be my last just for speaking here today," he added.

The prosecutor and policeman tried to defend themselves. They ended up blaming a militia in the area. They said they were work-ing to apprehend its members. But their words rang hollow. Each time they tried to defend themselves, the crowd scoffed at the ex-planations.

It became clear that the problem was not a lack of courage among the community, even less a lack of vigilance by the parents. Moth-ers and fathers described staying up all night. Some were exhausted from sleeping in shifts, taking turns to watch over their children. I was struck by the force with which many of the mothers spoke out.

The problem was the total lack of a functioning justice system. And this village outside Bukavu was a microcosm of our world. It might seem superficially far removed, with its wooden shacks and mud roads. Yet the problem the mothers of these girls faced was a problem faced by women everywhere: that even when they do speak up and denounce crimes against them, the criminal justice system so often fails them.

Sexual abuse thrives in silence, but it also thrives when men are free to act with impunity. Aristotle, the father of Western philoso-phy, wrote that "man, when perfected, is the best of animals. But when separated from law and justice, he is the worst of all." After everything that I have seen, I could not agree more.

In Kavumu, there were no laws; man was at his worst. But I witnessed, ultimately, just how powerful the justice system can be when sufficient resources and determination are brought to bear.

At the end of the meeting, several women and the community organizer who had spoken out in front of the crowd came to see me. In hushed voices that could not be overheard by others standing nearby, they told me who was ultimately responsible.

The militia active in the area was controlled by a local lawmaker, a member of the regional assembly in South Kivu. "Frederic Batumike. He's all-powerful. No one dares touch him," one of them said.

After the meeting, we stepped up our efforts to try to put an end to one of the most sickening sequences of attacks we'd ever known. In total, at least forty-six girls between eighteen months and ten years old were raped in Kavumu between 2012 and 2015.

We joined a broad coalition of actors that included the New York–based Physicians for Human Rights group, which I have worked with for more than a decade, as well as TRIAL International, a Geneva-based group focused on supporting victims through the judicial process. Our specialized legal team and doctors were essential.

In 2009, our Panzi Foundation created a new legal service as part of our "holistic care" program for survivors. It was a natural progression of our work, adding to the medical care, psychological support, and socioeconomic insertion programs run through the City of Joy and Maison Dorcas.

We noticed that many of the survivors who went through these programs overcame their injuries, rebuilt their confidence, and were ready to confront the stigmatization from their peers. With their sense of self-worth restored, they wanted to know how they could seek redress and justice, not just for themselves but so that others would avoid their fate.

When I see women ready to press charges, despite the low chances of success and the risk of intimidation, I know that the work of our teams is having an effect: it takes strength, belief in one's rights, and self-esteem, all things we try to encourage.

The legal arm of the hospital is known as the "judicial clinic" and was set up by an energetic lawyer, Thérèse Kulungu. Thérèse is from western Congo, but she volunteered to fly a thousand miles across the country to join us, having never set foot in Bukavu before, after reading about our work in the newspaper.

Her commitment has been matched by that of all of her successors, who oversee a team of six lawyers who help advise survivors on their legal rights. They assist them in lodging legal complaints and accompany them during trials. They also work with other lawyers and community leaders throughout the province, helping to educate citizens and women in particular about the criminal justice system.

It is essential and often dangerous work, which has been supported by several foreign partners, including the Eastern Congo Initiative, founded by actor Ben Affleck and Whitney Williams.

The work between the judicial clinic and the hospital's doctors, who have been trained in how to make forensic medical reports by Physicians for Human Rights, was vital in building up evidence against the perpetrators in Kavumu. We took detailed statements from victims and their families, recorded video interviews, and took photographs.

I also helped push media coverage in Congo and internationally. Belgian reporter Collette Braeckman was influential in Europe, while American journalist Lauren Wolfe wrote a detailed and moving story about Kavumu for *Foreign Policy* magazine in the United States, titled "A Miserable Mystery in Congo."

Pressure grew on the Congolese authorities to do something visibly. By then, Kabila's government had named a special representative for sexual violence, an act of window dressing rather than a real step to tackle the problem. When we contacted her about Kavumu, she said there was nothing she could do because of Batumike's parliamentary immunity as a member of the South Kivu assembly representing the area around Kavumu.

But the civilian prosecutor's office and police were ordered to step up their lackluster investigation in early 2016. Their efforts did not last long. Momentum soon stalled as they too concluded that Batumike could not be prosecuted.

Fortunately, the military justice system proved itself to be a more effective ally and less prone to corruption. In March, investigators from the military court in Bukavu assumed jurisdiction over the cases, arguing that the succession of rapes constituted a crime against humanity, which they had powers to prosecute.

Three months later, Batumike was arrested along with dozens of other men. He was detained at home, where police found an aging but still functioning semiautomatic Colt pistol stamped "U.S. Army," no doubt purchased on the huge black market for decommissioned weapons. This meant he could be charged with owning a weapon of war.

Investigators also found phone records showing him repeatedly in contact with several thugs from the militia who had been caught in the act of raping a young girl. They unearthed further links between him and the operational leaders of his armed group, which called itself Jeshi la Yesu (Jesus's Army). With this evidence, they were able to show that he was in control of these men.

The full story of their reign of terror came out when he and seventeen others were tried by the high military court in December 2017. Their grip on the area had begun when Batumike ordered the murder of a German expatriate who owned a plantation in the Kavumu area. The lawmaker had then tried unsuccessfully to seize his land. When he was denied the deeds for the property, he arranged for a group of men armed with Kalashnikovs to simply occupy the area.

The militia was then used to harass and silence anyone seen as a political opponent of the boss, including the murdered community organizer who had started investigating. Batumike was able to use his position, influence, and money to block police and judicial investigations against his henchmen.

The investigation shed light on the attacks on children. The court concluded that the fighters were under the sway of a witch doctor who prescribed potions that were supposed to protect them from their enemies. These concoctions required blood from the hymen of a virgin.

This sort of ritualistic quackery and superstition has a long history in Congo, although it does not normally involve sexual violence. It was famously part of the Simba rebellion against Mobutu in the 1960s, in which young fighters were administered black powder made from ground-up lion and gorilla bones and magic amulets that they believed turned enemy bullets into water.

During the three-week trial, the military court organized hearings in Kavumu where dozens of witnesses and victims came forward, many behind screens and with voice-altering technology to protect their identities—sadly, rare facilities in Congo. The mothers of the children were crucial. The vast majority stepped forward, telling of their horror and heartbreak and their fervent desire to see the men punished. In the final judgment, Batumike was sentenced to life in prison and eleven other members of the militia were convicted for crimes against humanity. It was the first time a sitting lawmaker in Congo had been found guilty for the crimes of his militia and the first conviction of sexual violence as a crime against humanity in a domestic court. The sentences were later upheld on appeal.

We were jubilant. The people of Kavumu were able to finally turn a page on five years of terror. Parents were able to sleep next to their children in peace. The rapes stopped just as suddenly as they had begun.

I haven't operated on a child from Kavumu since. There can be no stronger demonstration of the impact of justice.

Lawyers, doctors, and psychologists from the hospital continue to undertake risky missions to areas affected by mass rape in eastern Congo in order to take witness statements and prepare criminal complaints. These trips are arduous and often dangerous.

Once, a team found themselves stuck for several days on a jungle road waiting for help after their vehicle broke down. Sometimes they have to travel by boat up rivers and then walk for a whole day on jungle paths to reach the most remote villages. Everywhere they find survivors who dream of justice for their attackers but are skeptical about the chances and fearful for their own safety.

In late 2019, they scored another major success in helping with the prosecution of a warlord in the Shabunda region known as Kokodikoko. He led one of more than a dozen local so-called Mai-Mai militias, groups that supposedly defend the local population against Rwandan militants but in practice are brutal mafias involved in mining and extortion.

Military investigators, assisted by the UN, helicoptered in to put him on trial at the scene of many of the crimes, using a local church and a public building as makeshift courtrooms. There were 175 rape cases registered in the area. Along with our NGO partners and the UN, we helped secure witness protection measures that were vital to reassure women they would be secure if they testified.

In total, fifty victims came forward, including eight who had been abducted and kept as sex slaves in a cave by the militia. They knew the risk of reprisals if ever they were identified. But they also knew they were fighting for something bigger than justice for themselves. Their willingness to relive their experiences for the sake of justice helped protect others.

Kokodikoko, a former policeman turned gangster, was at first arrogant and contemptuous toward the court. He walked with a swagger and boasted that the trial was making him famous throughout Congo and overseas. He seemed to be reveling in the media attention. But he gradually lost his cool as the evidence mounted against him.

The court heard how he once kicked a man to death and how women, once captured, would be raped by him first, before being turned over to his men. At one point, Kokodikoko started to shout at the judges, his eyes bulging with anger, his face contorted with fury.

The testimony from witnesses and survivors, backed up by work from the Panzi team, was again essential in securing a life sentence for him and two other fighters for crimes against humanity. When he was convicted, he sobbed uncontrollably as he was led away in handcuffs.

In another first, the court also condemned the Congolese state for failing in its duty to provide protection for citizens who had appealed for help. The government was ordered to pay damages to the victims.

These are our success stories. They demonstrate that justice can be delivered with the help of a coalition of willing partners—medical, legal, and administrative—as well as a competent and reactive judicial authority. Both trials sent a message to commanders, politicians, and lowly foot soldiers that they might one day pay a price for their actions. These victories would have been impossible without brave and courageous survivors.

But, sadly, they are the exception.

The message over more than two decades to the war criminals in Congo is that they can continue massacring, torturing, raping, and looting without fear of the law or sanction. In many cases, such behavior is the route to power. There is a saying in Congo that to become a general in the army you need to have killed a thousand people. It remains a country of almost total impunity.

The caseload at our judicial clinic is constantly overwhelming, and the results are often dispiriting. In one recent case, a senior civil servant in Bukavu raped a girl in his car after a party. Despite overwhelming evidence against him, he secured his acquittal—reportedly for a fee of $10,000.

The civilian justice system is shot through with this sort of corruption when handling individual cases, even in cities like Bukavu. Convictions are for the poor; the powerful can almost always buy their freedom. Out in remote areas of eastern Congo, the police and the judicial system are often barely functioning even in government-controlled areas. Where rebel groups hold sway, proceedings are impossible.

The government at first denied there was a rape crisis and then became hostile to those of us who tried to tackle it, as I witnessed while being threatened in the Waldorf Astoria. There have been announcements, parliamentary investigations, and working groups looking into the problem of sexual violence, but there have never been the necessary reforms: funding and commitment to the domestic justice system, coupled with improvements to our dysfunctional security forces.

The two convictions secured against Batumike and Kokodikoko were possible only because of the exceptional reactivity of the military justice system and the rare application of international humanitarian law, which has expanded dramatically in the last two and a half decades.

Thanks to these advances, international law provides theoretical protections for women in conflict zones anywhere in the world. This represents progress, but again, the problem is one of implementation. The recent upsurge in nationalism globally is also undermining some of these cherished gains.

After World War II, the international tribunals set up to try war criminals—in Nuremberg, Germany, for Nazi atrocities in Europe and in Tokyo for the Asian violations—heard extensive evidence about the systematic use of rape, but they did not prosecute it as a crime against humanity. The Nuremberg trials did not prosecute rape at all.

In the 1990s, the first international tribunals since Nuremberg and Tokyo provided major leaps forward. At the International Criminal Tribunal for the former Yugoslavia, which sat in The Hague in the Netherlands from 1993, prosecutors for the first time demonstrated that rape could be considered a war crime and a crime against humanity.

In a landmark ruling in February 2001, the court successfully convicted three Serbian military and paramilitary figures who had raped non-Serb and Muslim women around the town of Foca in modern-day Bosnia and Herzegovina. They were sentenced to between twelve and twenty-eight years in prison for rape as a crime against humanity and for sexual slavery.

The International Criminal Tribunal for Rwanda, which opened in 1995 in Tanzania in East Africa, also established new jurisprudence on how rape could be prosecuted under international law. The case of Jean-Paul Akayesu, a Hutu mayor who directed the killing of up to two thousand people in his area, established for the first time that rape could amount to an act of genocide.

It is worth noting that the first charges brought against Akayesu did not include rape. Prosecutors either failed to identify or overlooked its widespread occurrence. The only female judge hearing the case, Navi Pillay from South Africa, was instrumental in admitting new evidence against him after a survivor gave excruciating testimony on the witness stand about the gang rape and abuse of Tutsi women in Akayesu's district. Pillay ordered that the charges be changed, a crucial example of a woman being more attuned and sensitive to the impact of sex crimes that her male colleagues had missed.

Akayesu was sentenced to life imprisonment in 1998.

These landmark judgments—that premeditated rape as a military tactic constituted a crime against humanity and a war crime and could be considered a method for committing genocide—were included in the founding treaty of the International Criminal Court. The creation of the ICC, which is also headquartered in The Hague in the Netherlands, was the high-water mark in the development of international humanitarian law. It was a landmark for humanity, a work of global cooperation, and a statement that the vilest acts of warfare would no longer be tolerated.

The ICC was created to be able to prosecute the world's most serious offenses—war crimes, crimes against humanity, and genocide—for atrocities committed after 2002, when it came into force. It was empowered to start investigations in countries that were either unwilling or unable to prosecute them. The message to warlords, dictators, and other human rights abusers was that nowhere offered them safety. Even failed states were no longer lawless territories.

Congo was among the more than 120 signatories of its founding treaty. This provided the legal basis for our military courts to prosecute Batumike and Kokodikoko. Without international humanitarian law, I might still be operating on young children from Kavumu.

In 2004, the government referred the conflict in eastern Congo to the ICC, where the chief prosecutor, Luis Moreno-Ocampo, duly opened an investigation. Where the national justice system had failed to punish offenders, perhaps international prosecutors could do better?

Congo was one of eight countries, all in Africa, where the ICC opened probes in its first decade of work. Moreno-Ocampo's decision to focus on Africa and not on other parts of the world was seen by some critics—mostly people with an ideological or personal interest in undermining his work—as an error of judgment.

There were isolated successes. In 2012, Thomas Lubanga, a militia leader active in the state of Ituri in eastern Congo who had links to Uganda, was found guilty of crimes against humanity for recruiting child soldiers as young as eleven for his group. It was the first successful conviction by the court and a reason to celebrate. But prosecutors overlooked widespread evidence of sexual crimes that might have increased the relatively lenient sentence of fourteen years' imprisonment. He has since been released.

In 2014, another militia leader active in Ituri, Germain Katanga, was sentenced to twelve years in prison over a village massacre. Sadly, he was acquitted of the charges of rape and sexual slavery.

In July 2019, there was a third victory: the ICC convicted Bosco

Ntaganda, a former general in the Congolese army turned rebel. He headed two Tutsi-dominated militias supported by Rwanda. The court heard how his men disemboweled babies, kept women as sex slaves, and beheaded civilians. He was found guilty of eighteen counts of war crimes, including rape, and sentenced to thirty years' imprisonment.

But these successes were rather like ours at a local level in the military courts: a proof of concept, a demonstration that the system could produce results. Yet they were entirely inadequate in creating the deterrence needed.

There are hundreds of men like these three high-profile convicts who have brought terror to the men, women, and children of eastern Congo. Some of them are in the army or working as businessmen in Congo or, like Laurent Nkunda, living in Rwanda, untroubled by the law.

And the ICC has come under sustained attack ever since its creation, including from the United States, which joined China and Israel in publicly voting against the creation of this vital supranational judicial body.

As the world's most powerful democracy, the United States should always be a champion of the rule of law. It was the driving force behind the multilateral international institutions set up after World War II. But the United States never signed up to the ICC, unlike all of its Western partners, putting it in a club of mostly authoritarian states who oppose it because they fear transparency and being accountable for their actions.

After the court's chief prosecutor tried to open an investigation in 2019 into war crimes committed in Afghanistan, an ICC member, the administration of U.S. President Donald Trump reacted with fury. The investigation will focus on Afghan government and Taliban crimes but also the well-documented torture and sexual abuse allegations against US forces during and after the 2003 invasion of the country. Trump announced sanctions targeting the chief prosecutor and another senior official.

The ICC has also been hit by threats of withdrawal from several

African countries, including Uganda, The Gambia, and South Africa, which have sought to portray the court as a conspiracy against the continent because of its early focus on Africa.

I don't deny that there are grounds to question the effectiveness of the ICC or its approach. For more than $1 billion in budget contributions, it has secured just nine convictions since 2002 and issued only thirty-five arrest warrants at the time of this writing. Several high-profile prosecutions have been bungled and mismanaged. But these failures should cause us to reflect on how to reform and improve this institution, not give in to pessimism and despair or conclude that the project is doomed. Many people have difficulty grasping the importance of multilateral institutions such as the ICC. They seem remote and complicated. They are under constant attack from nationalist politicians.

They are not perfect and must be constantly updated and improved. But their rules and regulations provide protection. Though it might seem irrelevant to Westerners with their well-funded justice systems, the ICC might be the only possible hope of redress for a Congolese mother who was raped daily in a forest camp or whose children were slaughtered in front of her. These are the human faces behind the laborious legal arguments and slow-moving trials in the courtrooms of The Hague.

Without the fear of paying a price for their actions, men will never be deterred from seeing women's bodies as objects to be seized, abused, and discarded in conflict zones. We will have no hope of making a rebel or army commander educate and discipline his soldiers. And I will have no hope of seeing an end to the constant stream of victims arriving at Panzi Hospital with their bodies torn and mutilated.

The total impunity with which crimes have been committed in Congo explains why they continue to occur today. It is why the former child soldier who spoke so shamelessly about his past in my office felt no fear in confessing to his crimes.

For this reason, I continue to plead for the international community to take action in all my public speeches, every time I accept an award on behalf of the battered women of Congo. It is incomprehensible to me why there has been no serious initiative to bring to justice the architects of Congo's suffering.

The genocides in the former Yugoslavia and Rwanda both gave rise to ad hoc international courts that together indicted more than 250 of the worst perpetrators. The Special Court for Sierra Leone, established in 2002, investigated the West African country's civil war in the 1990s and found former president Charles Taylor guilty of war crimes in 2012.

A criminal tribunal with international assistance was created in 2003 to prosecute the leaders of the Khmer Rouge in Cambodia who caused the deaths of more than 1.5 million people during a four-year period in the 1970s.

The death toll in Congo over two decades is gigantic. Again, as we do so often, we find ourselves short of exact data. Using excess mortality figures, the nonprofit International Rescue Committee calculated that as many as five million lives were lost directly through fighting, or from disease and malnutrition caused by the war, in just the first decade from 1998 to 2008. Yet other than the limited ICC investigations and occasional military trials in Congo, there has been no serious attempt to bring the creators of our misery to justice.

And it is not for lack of evidence. The Office of the UN High Commissioner for Human Rights undertook a detailed study of war crimes committed from 1993 to 2003, a period covering the two invasions of Congo by rebels backed by the armies of Rwanda, Uganda, and Burundi. More than twelve hundred eyewitnesses were interviewed by a team of more than twenty human rights experts.

It resulted in what is known as the Mapping Report,[1] a great slab of rigorous investigative work that runs to more than five hundred pages. It details 617 incidents of serious human rights abuses that could amount to crimes against humanity and possibly genocide, with the authors often grasping for the right language to describe what they refer to as "unspeakable cruelty."

Some of the incidents I was personally affected by: the attack on my hospital in Lemera features on page seventy-five; a massacre in my native village of Kaziba appears sixty pages later. A little further on, the report describes the massacre, mass rape, and mutilations in the village of Kasika, organized as revenge for an attack on rebel and Rwandan officers in August 1998.

One of the women killed was the pregnant wife of the tribal chief. I had examined her only weeks earlier and informed her she was expecting twins. She was disemboweled and had her babies ripped out of her womb. In the same region, in the center of the town of Mwenga, investigators discovered that fifteen women were raped, paraded naked through the streets, and then buried alive. There is horror on every page.

The UN commissioner responsible for the Mapping Report was Navi Pillay, the former South African judge who sat on the Rwandan genocide tribunal and made such a vital contribution to the definition of rape as a war crime. I count her among the many powerful women who have inspired me.

She was born in an Indian immigrant family in Durban and grew up in poverty before joining the anti-apartheid struggle. Through her determination and fierce intellect, she became the first nonwhite high court judge in her country. She is humble and uncompromising in her search for truth, and she conducts her work without fear or favor, earning herself many powerful enemies along the way.

The Mapping Report was the first attempt at accountability over the mayhem in Congo. When she published it in 2010, she was clear in linking the ongoing mass rapes and violence to judicial failings. "The culture of impunity in the DRC—which continues today— has encouraged the creation and evolution of armed groups and the use of violence to resolve disputes and gain control over natural resources," she stated.

For her efforts to shine a light on this shame, she was refused a second full term as commissioner and was pilloried by states hostile to the report, above all Rwanda. A draft was leaked to the press before publication, and media reports focused on the role of Rwanda's troops in the atrocities and the suggestion that their slaughter of Hutu refugees on Congolese territory could amount to genocide.

The Rwandan government "categorically rejected it" and said it was an attempt to "validate the double genocide theory," in which a second genocide took place against the Hutu inside Congo. President Paul Kagame, a former military commander, threatened to pull his country's three thousand peacekeepers out of UN operations. Secretary-General Ban Ki-moon made a rushed visit to the country to smooth over relations.

In the end, the final published version of the report was watered down. The word "allegedly" cropped up more frequently to imply doubt. And once it was released, it was filed away on a shelf or in a drawer somewhere in UN headquarters, where it remains to this day, more than ten years later, a colossal piece of work condemned to irrelevance.

The report made a series of recommendations, including that the government set up a credible "truth and reconciliation" mechanism to enable the country to confront its past and heal. It also suggested the creation of a special court composed of Congolese and international judges who would try the most serious human rights abusers. There were some suggestions at the time that the remit of the International Criminal Tribunal for Rwanda should be extended to prosecute crimes in Congo.

None of the recommendations were ever followed up on. President Joseph Kabila's desire to ignore it was simple to explain: He had served in his father's rebel group alongside Rwandan soldiers whose crimes had been documented. There was no appetite among world powers for pursuing the work of the Mapping Report either. The United States and the United Kingdom in particular continued to support and shield Rwanda. After being criticized for failing to foresee and prevent the genocide, the United States has poured tens of millions of dollars of humanitarian aid into Rwanda to help finance its reconstruction since 1994.

It remains highly sensitive and even dangerous to even raise the report and its recommendations internationally. On the occasion of its tenth anniversary in late 2020, I found myself the subject of a vicious smear campaign in state-run Rwandan media and received a flurry of new death threats after speaking out.

The international community continues to look the other way in Congo. There have been numerous other UN reports, such as those into the exploitation of Congolese raw materials, but little meaningful action beyond sending ever greater numbers of peacekeepers to try to keep a lid on the violence. Since 1999 there has been a UN peacekeeping force deployed in Congo that has steadily increased in size as the conflict has metastasized. It now numbers around sixteen thousand personnel and costs more than $1 billion a year, paid from UN funds to which the United States is the biggest contributor. It is the largest UN peacekeeping mission in history.

The police and soldiers who serve in Congo do their best with professionalism and courage. I am grateful to them for my own protection. Yet they are engaged in Congo in an unwinnable battle, too few to make an impact and with rules of engagement that prevent them from taking the fight to rebel groups.

Only justice and accountability can bring lasting stability to Congo, and rather than simply funding peacekeepers, the international community could use all of their leverage to bring the perpetrators to justice. Overall, the annual budget for the peacekeeping mission is eight times more than the budget for the International Criminal Court, with all of its investigations in multiple countries. It is a serious case of misplaced priorities.

The international community has never properly used all the levers at its disposal—legal, economic, and diplomatic—to bring an end to the conflict in Congo. The country is full of people ready to testify and longing for the day when the law overwhelms the gun as the foundation of authority. The women treated at my hospital are not crushed victims or mute casualties, silenced by the injuries inflicted on their bodies. They are courageous, powerful survivors prepared to speak up to help protect others.

But there needs to be a functioning justice system that can listen to them, put their tormentors behind bars, and send a message to others that the era of impunity has ended. The Congolese state should take the lead, of course. Since 2019, we have a new president who has promised to reform. But if Congo is unable to act, the ICC was created to step in for this purpose.

So far, I have dwelled on the mechanisms designed to bring perpetrators to justice in war zones where states often lack the means to bring rapists to justice. Now let us consider how sexual violence is prosecuted in peaceful countries. Are women better protected in places with functioning courts and police forces?

Sadly, the reality is not much different.

The US nonprofit Rape, Abuse & Incest National Network (RAINN) estimates that out of every 1,000 sexual assault cases, just 230 are reported to police.[2] A major survey based on interviews with forty thousand women by the European Union Agency for Fundamental Rights concluded in 2014 that across the twenty-eight-country bloc, only 14 percent of sex crimes were reported to the police.[3] The General Social Survey on Victimization in Canada of the same year concluded that just 5 percent of cases were reported.[4]

Sexual crime is the most underreported crime of all and, unlike other forms of violence, is not declining in developed countries, surveys have repeatedly shown. What's more, of the tiny minority of cases that are reported to law enforcement, only a fraction end up with a conviction. This is known as "attrition"—the number of cases that fail to result in a guilty plea or conviction.

For decades, feminist groups and governments have urged victims of sexual violence to find the courage to come forward and report their crimes. This was the subject of my last chapter. Breaking the silence and smashing taboos are essential if rape is to be meaningfully tackled.

The tragedy is that while in most countries women are heeding this advice in ever greater numbers, successful prosecutions have not risen in step. More and more are prepared to come forward. The #MeToo movement significantly boosted the trend.

Two researchers at Yale University looked at the number of reported cases in the world's thirty most developed countries in the six-month period after the first public allegations against Harvey Weinstein. The data showed an increase in reported sexual assault cases on average of 13 percent across all countries.[5]

However, in the United Kingdom the number of prosecutions has been falling in recent years in absolute terms. The Crown Prosecution Service in England and Wales brought charges in just 1,758 rape cases in 2018, down 38 percent from the year before.[6]

In France, #MeToo led to a surge in the number of cases being lodged, with a year-on-year increase of 11 percent in 2017, 19 percent in 2018, and 12 percent in 2019, according to figures from the Interior Ministry. Yet the trend for the number of convictions has been falling for the last decade. Between 2007 and 2017, the number of people convicted for rape fell by 40 percent.[7]

RAINN estimates that only 230 out of 1,000 rapes are reported to law enforcement in the United States. Out of the reported cases, 46 will lead to an arrest and only 5 will result in a conviction. That means that in 995 rape cases out of 1,000, the perpetrator gets away with it.

An analysis by *The New York Times* a year after #MeToo exploded in October 2017 found that a total of 201 men in prominent positions had been forced to resign following public allegations against them. More than half of them (124) were replaced by women, helping to address the huge gender imbalance in high-profile jobs. This is progress. But the number of prosecutions was still tiny.

Besides a handful of the most famous names—Weinstein, actor Bill Cosby, singer R. Kelly—very few were troubled by the arm of the law, as few as eleven according to an analysis by the *Axios* news site in March 2020.

For more women to speak out and report their experiences to the police, they must have confidence that the decision will be worth it. The problem is usually not the law itself. Advances in domestic legislation on sex crimes go back much further than the recent changes to international law, but they have the same flaw: they offer only theoretical protection.

The problem is the systemic biases that work against women in the criminal justice system. Much of this can be traced back to how rape has historically been prosecuted.

In the earliest civilizations, it was treated as a crime of adultery or fornication. Laws in medieval Europe evolved to consider rape a crime in its own right against women, but only if their "honor" had been impugned. Almost all legal systems included this concept as their central idea.

Only women who had honor in the first place—which excluded the poor, prostitutes, and minorities, for example—could be the victim of rape. And the all-male courts required women to prove that they were honorable.

Their sexual history became relevant evidence, as was any suggestion that they had somehow encouraged their attackers. Women were expected to have resisted the attack, because it was assumed that all "honorable" women would attempt to fight off their attackers to protect their reputations. An absence of injuries, or evidence that they had screamed for help, was therefore viewed as suspicious and disqualifying.

Unmarried women had to prove that they were virgins before the attack. Any previous sexual experiences would disqualify them as victims. Entirely unreliable so-called virginity tests—in which two fingers were inserted into their vaginas to test its elasticity— were commonplace in most European countries in the eighteenth and nineteenth centuries.

And all plaintiffs were viewed as inherently suspicious because it was widely assumed—by the male jurists—that women were prone to making up stories of sexual assault against men in order to force them into marriage or explain a pregnancy or because they were simply weak of mind and given to hysteria.

In seventeenth-century England, this was institutionalized with something called the "cautionary instruction," which was read out to juries before a trial, informing them that rape was an easy charge to make and difficult to defend against. The cautionary instruction spread throughout the British Empire and remained rooted in legal systems as far afield as Australia, the United States, Canada, a host of African nations, and Ireland until recently. Up until the 1970s and 1980s, judges would still inform juries that rape is a charge "easily made and, once made, difficult to defend against."

This very brief history lesson on how rape has been viewed and prosecuted is essential to understanding the biases and problems encountered today in Western legal systems. The notion of honor remains—a blunted, worn-down prejudice from a different era. It explains why prosecutors are unwilling to take on cases unless the woman is the "perfect victim," meaning she has no "disqualifying" characteristics, and why juries are so unwilling to convict.

High-profile cases in recent years involving victim blaming and efforts to cast women as being responsible for their assaults are a reminder that old habits and attitudes die hard. During the trial of Stanford University swimmer Brock Turner in 2016, his victim, Chanel Miller, was subjected to questioning from his defense attorney over her clothing, her relationship with her boyfriend, and her sexual history.

During the rape trial of two rugby players in a Northern Irish court in early 2018, the plaintiff's thong-style underwear was shown in court, which campaigners saw as a tactic to discredit her and a way of casting doubt on her character. Despite witness testimony that she was sobbing on the way home and a doctor's report observing a laceration to her vagina, the two sportsmen were acquitted.

In Spain, during the prosecution of four men who called themselves the "Wolfpack" in 2018, a lower-court judge admitted "evidence" from a private detective hired by one of the defendants that showed pictures of the teenage victim smiling with friends after her assault, as if to prove she was not traumatized.

All of these cases sparked protests, as much for the handling of the cases and treatment of the victims as for their final results. They showed that even in countries with some of the most protective laws, the sexism and bigotry rooted in centuries of discriminatory treatment of sexual assault victims continue to have an impact.

In other countries, survivors are still forced to undergo "virginity tests" on the basis that only sexual purity makes them reliable witnesses. According to UN Women, plaintiffs must undergo such tests in more than twenty countries, despite there being no medical basis for the procedure. In India, "two finger" testing was part of rape investigations until it was banned by the Supreme Court of India in 2013.

The idea that women are prone to lying remains deeply ingrained, even though there is no evidence to suggest that false rape allegations are a widespread problem. This is one of several rape "myths" that feminists have battled for decades. But everyone—from police officers, prosecutors, and judges to juries—is always on the lookout for the supposedly duplicitous woman.

Despite the intense media focus on occasional cases in which false allegations are proven or admitted to, all research suggests they are a tiny minority. The most commonly cited figures, based on three studies completed in the United States, put the number of "false" cases at somewhere between 2 and 10 percent, according to the US-based National Sexual Violence Resource Center. A major study by the Home Office in the United Kingdom in 2005 looked into 3,527 rape cases lodged with law enforcement and concluded that only 9 percent were "determined to be false."[8]

We must be aware of these historic biases against sexual assault survivors in order to understand why, after half a century of huge progress in widening and improving legislation, reporting and convictions remain so shockingly low.

Laws against sexual assault and harassment have been greatly expanded since the 1970s thanks to the efforts of feminist organizations. Sexist language that refers to the honor, chastity, or modesty of a woman has been stripped out. Marital rape has become a crime, overturning the notion that the marriage contract was the granting of permanent sexual consent.

The notion of what rape entails has also been widened to include the unwanted penetration of any orifice, not just the vagina, which provides theoretical protection for male victims, too. Unwanted penetration with fingers or any other objects can be prosecuted in the same way as penetration with a penis.

So-called rape shield laws have greatly restricted the use of the sexual history of the victims to discredit them. There is no longer any emphasis on the need for physical injuries to prove an allegation, recognition that many victims simply freeze out of fear or can be coerced into sex against their will. And victims are no longer forced to report their assault to authorities immediately afterward—another discriminatory aspect of early rape laws.

The most advanced legislation in the world today is based on consent. It removes any need for a jury or judge to consider whether there was physical violence. It simply demands that consent must be freely granted by both partners and that certain individuals—the unconscious or vulnerable, for example, or anyone being threatened or coerced—are unable to give it.

Sweden made headlines in 2018 when it went further than most with a new rape law that requires both partners to give explicit approval for sex, either verbally or physically. This is the "yes means yes" model, unlike other laws that require a partner to have refused consent ("no means no") for the penetration to be considered rape.

It led to exaggerated reports and mockery from some conservatives that lovers in Sweden would now need to sign contracts before going to bed or would have to put aside their passion to pause for a discussion about whether they both consented. The key and admirable point of this law is the message it sends: that both partners, but particularly women, have to actively demonstrate or verbalize their approval at all stages. The problem is that "consent" is still misunderstood by large numbers of people.

In other countries, the advances in women's rights have stalled or never taken place. It is not a simple picture of backward developing countries and more advanced Western ones. Malta, for example, a small but wealthy EU member in the Mediterranean, still considered rape a crime "affecting the good order of families" until 2018. Congo has had an excellent law on rape since 2006, but the problem, as with so much Congolese legislation, is implementation.

In a major review of sexual assault legislation in eighty-two jurisdictions published in 2018, the US-based campaign group Equality Now highlighted how in at least nine countries, including Iraq, Kuwait, and the Philippines, it was still possible to escape punishment for rape if the perpetrator married the victim. Lebanon, Jordan, and Tunisia had similar laws that were changed only in 2017.

Married women in countries as diverse as Singapore, India, and Sri Lanka could not be raped by their husbands because marital rape was not a recognized offense. Dozens of others had old-fashioned language or required evidence to be presented in court, which made it all but impossible to secure convictions. In Senegal in West Africa, rape was not considered a serious offense until January 2020, when it was reclassified as a felony rather than a misdemeanor.

The first step to tackle the global rape epidemic is having clear legislation, using the concept of consent, that fully recognizes women as autonomous, independent individuals. Strict sexual assault laws with long prison sentences for rape act as both a deterrent and, when drafted, an opportunity to educate men and women about their rights and responsibilities.

But this is only the beginning, as Congo's law in 2006 shows. Unless it is considered part of a much broader set of reforms, which require resources and education, then the law alone will never succeed in making a meaningful impact.

There are many things that can be done. The most radical campaigners have suggested reversing the "presumption of innocence" principle for sexual assault cases, meaning the accused would be assumed to be guilty unless he could prove his innocence. It would lead to miscarriages of justice for sure, but perhaps at a lower rate than presently, when most rapists walk free.

I can see the appeal of the arguments but do not agree. We must look at how to improve the current system, making it fairer and more balanced in how it responds to allegations of rape, rather than overturning foundational legal principles.

The most important area to focus on is the provision of trained staff who can help orient victims when they seek assistance or advice. These first conversations usually take place at either a hospital or a police station and are absolutely crucial in determining whether a woman decides to lodge a complaint.

Nurses, doctors, and law enforcement officers need to know how to look for and preserve evidence that can be used for a future prosecution. This means testing for DNA contained under fingernails, on skin, or inside the body, as well as examining the individual for signs of injury consistent with rape. They need to make detailed written statements and establish a medical certificate that can be admitted in court.

All of this, through force of habit, we do at Panzi Hospital every time we receive a new patient, but these routines and practices are not commonplace in medical institutions and police forces that have not been sensitized to the specific requirements of handling sexual assault crimes. A major cultural shift is required, particularly in workplaces where ignorance, sexism, and misogyny are commonplace. The work is procedural and administrative, but there is also an important psychological and social dimension.

It is vital that a police officer or nurse receiving a sexual assault victim understands the person's sense of vulnerability, and potentially shame, about what has happened to her. A badly formulated question ("Are you sure it's true that . . .") or an unsympathetic attitude ("Why did you agree to meet him?") can reinforce the common feeling among victims that they were in some way responsible for the crime against them.

Medical and law enforcement staff also need to understand the consequences of trauma, which can often have an impact on a victim's ability to recall details and recount events in a chronological order. Many patients have told me how they lost consciousness or simply froze and felt an almost out-of-body experience, which leaves them with only hazy memories of their attacker. These are not signs that should arouse suspicion.

The provision of specialized female police officers trained in handling sexual assaults can help to improve the reporting of sex crimes and convictions. Women generally feel more comfortable talking about intimate sexual experiences with another woman, an issue for police forces that are male-dominated worldwide.

The idea of "one stop" centers for victims of sexual assault, where police and medical personnel as well as psychological counselors are available twenty-four hours a day, has also gained momentum. The first centers like these were opened in the United States in the 1970s and have expanded since. The United Kingdom and Canada have similar publicly funded initiatives, while Belgium and France are in the process of expanding their own versions of the same concept. The Indian government, too, made creating rape crisis centers part of its response to the 2012 New Delhi gang rape that sparked protests.

They are a vital resource for the people who use them and may play an important role in disseminating knowledge in the population and in law enforcement communities. But unless their existence is widely publicized, these advantages are lost. The other problem is one of scale: they are usually viable only in major population centers and are frequently underresourced.

The longer-term solution is one of sensitizing all police and medical services, from rural areas to major cities, making them aware and prepared when a woman steps forward with allegations of sexual assault. Because of the sheer pervasiveness of the myth that women are prone to making up vindictive sexual assault allegations, law enforcement officials often fail to act or conduct shoddy investigations in which evidence is missed. This still happens almost everywhere. Too many police officers either don't care about or actively uphold the culture of violence against women.

Because of my expertise I am occasionally called upon to advise on cases overseas requiring particularly complex reconstructive surgery, and I operated on a patient in Belgium a few years ago.

This patient was suffering from a traumatic fistula, inflicted during a gang rape, which had relapsed despite several rounds of surgery.

We succeeded in treating her, but I was shocked to learn afterward about her experience with the police. When she went to her local station to report the crime in a state of profound shock, she was treated as if she were drunk. She was taken to a cell to sober up. Only later did officers notice her bleeding and take her to the hospital.

The city of Detroit provided a tragic example of what happens when a police force fails to take investigating sex crimes seriously. In 2009, more than eleven thousand rape kits that are used to gather DNA after an attack were discovered in a decrepit city warehouse. They had never been tested.

The invention of the first rape kit, a collection of vials and swabs for collecting forensic evidence, was credited in a recent investigation by *The New York Times* to an entirely overlooked and forgotten activist and campaigner in Chicago in the 1970s named Marty Goddard.

Marty was appalled by the lack of effort in investigating rape cases and how officers routinely destroyed evidence. At the time, the Chicago police training manual informed new officers that "many rape complaints are not legitimate" and that an "actual rape victim will generally give the impression of a person who has been dishonored."[9]

The discovery of the abandoned Detroit kits caused a scandal and led to the opening of hundreds of investigations over the last ten years. There were several thousand matches in the FBI's forensic database. As a result, more than eight hundred suspected rapists were identified, resulting in nearly two hundred convictions by the end of 2019.[10] Several of these identified rapists had gone on to assault other victims in the years that rape kits holding their DNA languished untested.

When campaigners talk about the need for "systemic" change to the criminal justice system, this is what they mean: unless you change the whole system so that every part works, you won't get results. One weak link in the chain can doom a woman's chances of getting justice and condemn others to being future victims.

Look at the Detroit example: the city was covered by the state of Michigan's strict consent-based rape law that punishes sexual assault with up to life imprisonment; the police force had been equipped with rape kits to take evidence; thousands of women heeded the advice of campaigners and came forward to lodge cases and give DNA.

Consider the amount of work required to get to this point. It was the result of literally decades of investment from legislators and civil society groups. But their efforts went to waste because frontline police officers could not be bothered to process evidence and investigate properly.

Sadly, most women around the world do not have access to rape kits and must deal with police officers who are untrained in how to conserve evidence in a rape case or are hostile to doing so. And unless a victim is examined medically within seventy-two hours of a sexual assault, any physical evidence that can be gathered is likely to have been lost.

The understandable impulse for many victims is to destroy all memories of the encounter with their rapist. I have known some who have burned their clothes, while others have told me they showered repeatedly afterward to try to get rid of the smell of their attacker.

Another area that requires attention is the statute of limitations on sexual assault cases. It varies from country to country and sometimes within them. The idea of putting a time limit on how long a crime can be prosecuted after the fact is intended to balance the need for upholding the law against the danger of laying charges against someone based on recollections that have faded and changed over time.

Yet in most countries there is no limitation for murder, considered the most serious of crimes. Why treat rape differently, when we know of its devastating impact? In the United States, for example, Alaska has no time limit on prosecuting rape, while Massachusetts has a fifteen-year cutoff.[11]

Sex crimes are different from other felonies. They can take years to process before a victim feels comfortable and confident about coming forward, particularly if the abuse occurred as a child or was perpetrated by a family member. These factors argue in favor of long statutes of limitations.

And in cases when DNA is collected afterward, why should this evidence be seen as out of date if a match is found twenty or even thirty years later?

The scale of sexual abuse in conflicts and in peacetime, coupled with the difficulty in collecting evidence and the lack of witnesses, makes it tempting for some people to think it is a problem that can never be eradicated. So often the pessimists will say sex crimes are impossible to prosecute, that the cases amount to one person's word against another's—"she said versus he said"—for crimes that usually take place behind closed doors.

They are wrong. There are a host of ways that governments can improve how evidence is collected and investigations are carried out. It does require sustained investment and resources, I do not deny it.

But let us try to imagine a type of crime that women overwhelmingly inflicted on men. Let's say, for the sake of argument, that a scourge of painful and violent penis assaults emerged that caused men serious psychological distress and sometimes physical injuries.

The problem became so serious that thousands of men came forward with allegations, yet the police were uninterested in investigating. A few cases came to court, but the accused women all walked free. The men had hurt themselves, judges or juries concluded. Hearing more and more reports of attacks, all men started to feel vulnerable.

It is inconceivable that this would not be treated as a scandal. There would be demonstrations in the streets. Politicians would outdo each other with promises of "exemplary justice" for the guilty, tougher sentences, and extra resources for education and investigations. Newspapers would run campaigns pushing for action. In chapter 3, I told you about the case of a young male patient in 2008 whose penis had been cut off. The extraordinary press interest in his case, even though my wards were full of injured women, could not have been a clearer demonstration of the gender biases in media coverage.

The level of sexual crime against women across the world is a real scandal, not an imaginary one. It is happening right now. It continues because of sexism and the lack of value placed on women's lives. It should be a national security priority in every country.

For everyone who doubts that justice can be delivered, I refer them to our case against Batumike in Kavumu. Prosecutors and police insisted that he was untouchable, that nothing could be done. He is now behind bars and will remain there, God willing, for the rest of his life.

We need more victories like this in Congo, Myanmar, Sudan, Syria, Iraq, Yemen, and Afghanistan, not less. We need more international justice and cooperation among nations to support the rule of law. We need more men like Weinstein behind bars.

Punishing rapists and sexual abusers sends the message that sexual assault is unacceptable. Convictions educate and deter. Everywhere that men behave as "the worst of all" animals, on battlefields or in bedrooms, they must know that they risk ending up in court.

8

RECOGNITION AND REMEMBRANCE

*I*t is hard to overstate the importance of improving the way our criminal justice and international judicial systems handle complaints about sexual violence. There is so much work to be done in making them more responsive, sensitive to victims, and effective in putting rapists behind bars. Yet in some cases, when identifying the attacker is near impossible or evidence cannot be collected—in a war zone, for example—we have to think about how women can be recognized or compensated using other methods.

In 2010, I flew to a region that I had heard so much about but never visited. It had been described to me during bedside visits at the hospital or in my consulting room, often through tears, by my patients. It was a place that had become associated in my mind with the worst sorts of abuses, poverty, and official neglect that are such features of life in eastern Congo.

Since the opening of our hospital in Panzi in 1999, there had been a constant stream of girls and women from the region of Shabunda, some who had made the two-hundred-mile trip under their own steam, others who were deposited semiconscious or dying by relatives or aid agencies. Collectively, they had left a mark on the hospital and on me, none more than Wamuzila, whom I described in chapter 4, or the girl who caused the general to faint at the hospital in 2006, which I wrote about in chapter 6.

The communities in Shabunda, like every one in eastern Congo, have been failed by the army, which has been unable to root out the armed groups that cause constant dread and pain. They have been failed by the justice system, meaning rapists and killers continue to act without fear of the law. And they have been let down by the state, which fails to provide basic services such as water, electricity, or maintenance on the only road linking the region to the outside world.

The whole area is around the size of the state of Vermont or slightly smaller than Belgium, with a population estimated at about a million people. It is covered by the dense equatorial forest that blankets most of Congo. I observed and admired the canopy as I flew there on a UN helicopter from Bukavu.

Viewed from the air, our jungle looks like a gigantic field of tightly packed heads of broccoli crammed together as far as the eye can see, an immensity of greenness that obscures the earth and ground below. I imagined the undergrowth beneath this thick layer of leaves and branches fighting for light, the dappled shade, the footpaths cut through vines, and the sound of birdsong. It was the kind of wilderness I once loved walking in but am barely ever able to appreciate nowadays.

It was easy to see why Shabunda had become such a formidable redoubt for the guerrilla groups that have terrorized the area and its inhabitants since the late 1990s. The inhospitable forest, its caves, and the rocky outcrops provide perfect hiding places for those prepared to endure the hardships of poor diet, mosquitoes, and snakebites.

Down below the leaves, I knew there were the rebel camps where men were milling around, perhaps plotting another nighttime raid that would spill more blood. How many women were being held at gunpoint at the very moment I swooped overhead?

There were signs of the illicit activity that fuels the fighting as I flew toward the main town in Shabunda. Every once in a while, the dense foliage would give way, as if a great paw had scraped back the wilderness to reveal deep red scars of mud and mounds of earth. The trees had been cleared, not with one great sweep but with thousands of strokes from hand-pulled saws, ancient woodland pulled down with ropes and grunts.

On the exposed parts of the ground, I could see men and boys working below, tiny, almost naked figures entering rathole mines or hacking away at the surface, shovels and plastic bowls in hand as they hunted for the coltan, gold, or tin buried beneath. In which products, where in the world, would the fruit of their labor end up? They looked up and stared blankly.

At other points, in the shallow edges of streams and rivers, small groups could be seen bent over, ankle-deep in muddy brown water, panning for flakes of gold in the sediment. I would point them out to my fellow travelers, gesturing with my hand and doing my best to shout above the din of the rotors.

I was on a fact-finding mission funded by the Office of the UN High Commissioner for Human Rights. It was led by Deputy Commissioner Kang Kyung-wha from South Korea and included former Finnish defense minister Elizabeth Rehn, as well as a senior UN official from New York and women's rights activist Jessica Neuwirth, who would become a firm friend during our work together. We had been asked to meet victims of sexual violence in Congo and examine their needs in terms of reparations.

We had been tasked with evaluating the performance of the justice system, which I knew was nearly nonexistent, but more important to look into the question of how victims might be compensated in other ways for their suffering.

It was often heartbreaking work, but it revealed to me an important truth: not only does the justice system fail survivors of sexual violence but governments compound this shortcoming by failing to acknowledge survivors in different ways that can help alleviate their suffering.

We landed at an airstrip in the main town of the Shabunda region, which is also called Shabunda. Almost all the goods required by the local population arrive here on this bumpy landing strip, which is just long enough for small planes to arrive laden with refreshments, kitchen utensils, batteries, or medicine. As a result of the scarcities, a bottle of water or Coke in Shabunda can cost as much as in a Western capital.

There was a welcome party of dozens of people whose songs we could hear faintly as the helicopter engine wound down. Most of them were women and they surged forward as we stepped down from the aircraft, its blades swinging in ever-slowing circles over our heads.

I embraced as many of them as I could. It was an emotional reunion with patients who had spent time at the hospital, many of whom I had operated on personally. I recognized a few faces. I had never set foot here before, but the broad smiles and hugs made it feel like a homecoming.

A local high-ranking official was there to greet us, too, as was the commander of the local battalion of UN peacekeepers. They both gave us an update on the security situation, explaining that the area was safe around the town, which was home to about twenty thousand people; but beyond this perimeter, the army and UN were unable to guarantee security to the inhabitants.

There had been an upsurge in attacks in the territory over the last month, we were told. Peacekeepers would travel to the scene when they could, but even they found it difficult to reach some of the villages. There were vast areas that were simply inaccessible by road and too dangerous to reach by air.

Accompanied by a crowd of local women and the official, and escorted by UN peacekeepers, we were led to the middle of the town to a statue that had been erected in tribute to the survivors of the area. It was as unexpected as it was inspiring.

Cast in bronze and atop a concrete plinth, it depicted a woman on her haunches. The figure had one arm stretching behind her, with her hand touching the ground to support her weight; her other hand was clasped to her forehead. Her head was cast back, her face tilted toward the sky, and her features bore the stricken expression of someone coming to terms with a sudden, unforeseen pain. In her pose, she looked weighed down by physical agony but still, it seemed to me, strong enough to struggle back to her feet.

It was unsettling to behold, but immensely powerful in what it captured and symbolized. Our guides explained that the statue had been placed facing eastward toward Congo's neighbors, Rwanda in particular, which the community viewed as the source of their misfortune and fear.

We moved on and were led to a building in the town where we had arranged to sit down with survivors who had agreed to talk to us about their experiences on this leg of our journey. In total, we held meetings in seven different places around the country, with each stop a lesson in the barbarism of the conflict and the courage of its victims.

Although each person was told that she was not obliged to describe her experience and that our intention was to learn about the women's needs, all offered their personal stories unprompted, often explaining that they wanted the world to know about what was happening.

We met a couple who had been attacked by Mai-Mai militants in their village in 2005. The wife had been gang-raped and left with deep pink disfiguring scars on her leg where she had been set on fire. Her husband, who had tried to come to her rescue, had been beaten nearly to death, losing twelve teeth and most of his hearing in the process.

He recounted how friends and family had encouraged him to abandon his wife after the attack, but he had decided to stand by her and their six children. He understood that it was not her fault, providing a rare and uplifting example of a couple facing adversity together. Most others did not benefit from supportive spouses.

All seven of the survivors stressed that the most important response to their suffering would be bringing peace and security to the region so that others would avoid their fate. "What bothers me most is that our enemies are still there," one of them told us. "Even if we got help individually, if our enemies are still around, there will be no end to our problems." Others made practical suggestions such as bringing water points closer to villages so that girls would not have to venture far to fetch water from wells or streams. Justice, too, was important, even though few voiced any hope of seeing their tormentors on trial.

But our final encounter that day left a profound effect on me. It made me realize how the failure to publicly acknowledge sexual violence in conflicts has an impact on victims. Our final interview was with the oldest woman we met in Shabunda, a sixty-one-year-old widow who had been abducted for six days and gang-raped in the jungle.

She was powerfully built and spirited. She sat with us in her beautiful patterned *pagne,* her head held high and defiantly. She began by telling us about her experience, and once she had finished, I asked what she needed.

"I don't need anything," she replied. Her eyes flashed with indignation. "But I want one thing. We women deserve respect.

"We give birth, we bring up children, we work. But we are being humiliated. I was humiliated by children, the same age as my grandchildren. Nothing can remove this shame, nothing. But what I want is for the president to come here and apologize in public.

"I want him to come and recognize our suffering and the crimes against us. That would help me heal, that would make me feel respected again by people here," she said.

I looked at her with profound admiration. There was such wisdom and strength in what she said. Like almost all of the survivors we met, she did not yearn for revenge. In the overwhelmingly majority of cases, the women wanted peace, schools to educate their children, or new churches to help bring the community back together.

But the elderly widow had struck upon something essential that is often withheld from women who suffer from the sexual violence: recognition. She wanted to be acknowledged and to hear an apology for the failure to protect her. She didn't want it only for herself: she wanted it for others like her who continued to suffer in silence.

Yet this sort of recognition is so rarely offered. In Congo, during his time in office from 2001 to 2019, President Kabila did the opposite. He denied and obfuscated; he threatened people like me who tried to draw attention to the crisis. He refused to fund public compensation schemes that would have paid reparations to these women.

The statue of the survivor on her haunches in the center of the village was part of the process of recognizing the women of Shabunda. It was the first time I had ever seen a public tribute to the women victims of Congo's wars. Nothing like it exists in Bukavu.

The women we interviewed said they admired it. It helped lift the sense of shame some of them still felt. Its existence sent a message that they were worthy of admiration and sympathy, rather than the stigmatization they so often suffered from.

It set me wondering how many statues or tributes to the rape victims of other conflicts have been erected around the world. For World Wars I and II, almost every French and British village will have some sort of monument to commemorate the fallen and injured soldiers during the battles of those awful conflicts. Politicians pay tribute to their bravery in annual ceremonies. Let us never forget their sacrifices, people are told—and rightly so.

But who remembers the hundreds of thousands, perhaps millions, of women who were also victims, raped at the barrel of a gun by German, Russian, or Allied troops, or coerced into sex in order to save themselves or their families? Who remembers the children born out of these forced relationships?

The instinct to cover up abuse at the individual level, in which women are told not to make a fuss and that their experience is something shameful, operates at the institutional and governmental levels as well. Women's experience of war and conflict is different. They are rarely combatants and almost never the initiators, but the toll on them is no less significant.

It seems to me that part of the problem is how we record armed conflicts, which has an influence on how we then recall and commemorate them. The first draft of history is written by journalists, which makes the gender imbalance in the world's media, historically and still today, part of the reason women find themselves so often literally written out of the past.

Since 1995, the Global Media Monitoring Project has conducted reviews of the world's print and broadcast media to check the representation of women. It has conducted five studies since then, the last in 2015. They show precious little change over this twenty-year period. Only 24 percent of news subjects—the people who are interviewed or whom the news is about—are female.

Men make up most of the journalists worldwide, and their dominance is particularly marked in the senior editor jobs that set the news agenda. They also have a near monopoly in the specialized realm of war reporting. On assignment, women reporters face additional dangers of harassment and assault, but their perspective and ability to speak to and gain the trust of fellow women are often essential in capturing their stories.

Once the journalists have done their work, those responsible for creating the successive drafts of history also tend to be male. History departments skew male in most universities, and popular senior historians—who write the landmark studies and best-selling books on conflicts—are for the most part men, too.

Accounts of war tend to focus on the strategic decision-makers, battlefield action, technological progress, troop losses and injuries, and individual acts of valor. At every stage, the politicians, tacticians, commanders, and soldiers are men. This is how wars are portrayed in films and children's schoolbooks, too. Women barely get a look at, other than as collateral damage.

A few years ago, I read a book coauthored by Rochelle G. Saidel, an American academic and founder of the Remember the Women Institute, which helped change my perspective on World War II. In the late 1970s, she became interested in sexual abuse during the Holocaust because of a Nazi war criminal hearing that took place in the United States in Albany, New York, where she was living at the time.

She met some of the female witnesses who had been flown over from Israel by the US government to testify during a deportation hearing against a Latvian man, Vilis Hāzners, who had been an officer in Adolf Hitler's Waffen-SS. Listening to the stories, she became

Fulton County Library System

Customer Name: Miller, Melody Nashelle
Customer ID: D025934555

Items that you checked out

Title: The power of women : a doctor's journey
of hope and healing
ID: R4003979460
Due: 12/29/2021 11:59 PM

Total items: 1
Account balance: $0.00
12/15/2021 2:49 PM
Checked out: 1
Overdue: 0
Hold requests: 0
Ready for pickup: 0

Thank you for using the bibliotheca SelfCheck
System.
www.afpls.org

inspired to investigate the incidence of sexual violence during the Holocaust, something that was barely ever talked about.

She began researching, examining archival writings and documents, and conducting interviews with survivors. She visited Ravensbrück, a Nazi concentration camp for women in eastern Germany. She also teamed up with Dr. Sonja Hedgepeth, a fellow academic with the same interests as her.

There was a lack of documentation about sexual crimes during the Holocaust, but not because it did not exist. Nazi racial laws strictly forbade relationships and physical contact with Jews. As a result, there was almost nothing recorded. Yet a system of brothels and sexual slavery thrived in detention and forced labor camps. As they unearthed more evidence of widespread sexual abuse, Saidel and Hedgepeth began running workshops to spread awareness about Jewish women's experiences. During one of them at Yad Vashem, the World Holocaust Remembrance Center in Jerusalem, a highly respected Israeli scholar of the period was among the audience.

During their presentation, when Saidel mentioned mass rape, he stood up and interrupted them, visibly angry. "Jewish women were not raped during the Holocaust. Where are the documents?!" he shouted.[1] They realized that they were challenging one of the last taboos of this most infamous period of the twentieth century.

The two professors decided it was time to write a book to challenge the orthodox view that sexual violence had not featured during the Holocaust. By denying or ignoring it, historians were depriving women of the recognition they deserved. The result of their work, the first of its kind, was published in 2010 under the title *Sexual Violence Against Jewish Women During the Holocaust*.

The reason so little had been written about the sexual abuse of Jewish women was the reason so little is known about sexual violence all over the world. Survivors were fearful of the personal cost of speaking out, of being stigmatized by their community.

Many were young women at the time of the abuse who worried about their marriage prospects as a rape survivor after the end of the war. But they also had an additional pressure that is unique to the Holocaust: because of the mind-numbing scale of the killing and torture, they felt that raising sexual violence might detract somehow from the losses suffered by others. If they were alive to denounce sex crimes at the hands of Nazi soldiers or fellow prisoners, then they were more fortunate than their six million fellow Jews who had been murdered.

Another reason many survivors had not spoken out, which is highly relevant to my point about female representation in the fields of the media and history, was that no one had spent time looking for them and persuading them to share their memories until Rochelle Saidel and Sonja Hedgepeth came knocking.

None of the (almost entirely male) reporters, historians, and prosecutors who helped reveal the full extent of the concentration camps and state-sponsored killing ever went looking for evidence of sexual violence. They didn't find it because they never asked, or they never asked in a way that was likely to elicit deeply personal admissions. As I mentioned in the last chapter, the Nuremberg trials for Nazi criminals did not prosecute anyone for rape or sex crimes.

For the survivors, the emotional cost of suppressing their memories can be measured by an interview Saidel conducted with a social worker at a nursing home in Toronto that cared for Holocaust survivors. The social worker told her that very often dying women would need to get something off their chest before they breathed their last.

"I need to tell you something," they'd say as their lives slipped away. "I was raped, but don't tell my family."[2]

Reading about these women breaks my heart. All their lives they concealed their pain, their inner damage, feeling either ashamed or unworthy of attention and sympathy. Only on their deathbeds did they liberate themselves from the burden of secrecy.

As a result of Saidel and Hedgepeth's work, attitudes have started to change. Male scholars no longer interrupt their speeches and seminars. In 2018, they organized a trailblazing exhibition,

VIOLATED: Women in Holocaust and Genocide, at the Ronald Feldman Gallery in New York that showcased art depicting sexual abuse during World War II, in Rwanda, and in Bosnia.

Admitting the existence of sexual violence has not detracted from the sickening reality of the ghettos or the gas chambers. It has contributed to a more inclusive account of what happened. The recognition came too late for the poor women of the Toronto nursing home whose final words were a whispered confession, but it should make us reflect on the gender biases contained in our common human history.

In 2018, I flew halfway across the world to meet another group of women whose fight for recognition has made them heroes in their country and far beyond. They have achieved more than anyone else in teaching the world about the damage of sexual violence in conflict and the importance of expressing remorse. In my conversations with them, I found echoes of what I had heard from the elderly widow I had encountered in Shabunda whose greatest desire was for an apology from President Kabila.

They are South Korea's "comfort women," and they represent the estimated two hundred thousand girls and young women who were forcibly recruited and trafficked as sex slaves for use by the Imperial Japanese Army during its military campaigns in Asia from the start of the twentieth century until its defeat in 1945. I prefer their Korean name, *halmoni,* which translates as "grandmothers."

Their story—of broken lives and decades of silence—inspires pity, but their campaign for a formal apology and acceptance of responsibility from the Japanese state deserves our profound admiration. Carried out with quiet dignity and steely determination, their struggle right into the final years of their lives is motivated by a desire to heal personally but also by the conviction that they are helping others.

As a result of their campaign, which has caused major diplomatic tensions with Japan, South Korea is perhaps one of the most sensitized countries in the world to the issue of sexual violence in conflict. Their suffering has been repeatedly acknowledged by their own government, and they have statues and a museum dedicated to their lives.

The War and Women's Human Rights Museum was one of my first stops in Seoul, the first museum of this kind that I had ever visited. It's a modest building in a residential backstreet that took years to build because of wrangling over its location. Some Korean veterans' associations objected to initial plans to house it in a park in Seoul honoring "martyrs" of the country's independence fight, as if raped women would somehow sully the memory of the liberation movement.

What the museum lacks in size it makes up for in impact. Over its two floors, and a dimly lit and empty concrete basement meant to convey the grim and disorienting conditions in which many women were kept, visitors learn the true horrors of what befell those who were abducted and then imprisoned in state-sanctioned brothels.

I was struck by a wall featuring concrete molds of the faces and hands of some of the grandmothers. They look as if they are pushing through the surface, symbolizing the difficulty of breaking the veil of silence and going public with their experiences. Another wall is composed of bricks, each with a picture and message from a different survivor, with holes left for those who were never able to come forward.

I stopped and stared at a photograph of a miserable-looking, stick-thin young woman being inspected by a Japanese doctor in a white medical coat. I wondered how this doctor could betray his education and the ethics of my profession in the service of such abominable cruelty. Once abducted, each woman had to undergo regular, humiliating checks for sexually transmitted diseases.

I left feeling outraged and humbled as I headed to a residence in the capital where a dwindling group of grandmothers live together and are cared for. I met Kim Bok-dong, then ninety-one, an elegant but frail survivor with gray hair that framed her gentle face. She spoke to me quietly and gravely of her experiences, as well as her hopes for what little time remained of her life.

Kim was fourteen when soldiers showed up at her house in Yang-san in the south of the country during the occupation of South Korea by Japan. Her parents were told that she was needed to work in a factory as part of the war effort, a demand they knew they were unable to refuse. With Japan then at war with China, Koreans were being forcibly recruited into the military.

Kim was plucked from her home and found herself the youngest in a group of other women all around eighteen to twenty years old. They were packed into a truck and taken to a nearby port at the start of a journey that would see them transported like cattle, via several different ships, to their destination in Guangdong Province in southern China, which was also under Japanese occupation. Along the way, she had no idea where she was heading. She felt like any fourteen-year-old would—insecure and homesick—and she knew nothing of her captors' intentions.

Once she landed in Guangdong, she was taken to a Japanese military facility, an occupied factory building, where she was examined physically and then put to work. She was beaten by the first soldier who raped her. The experience was excruciating.

She tried to commit suicide along with two other women. Her mother had given her some money as a leaving present, which she had managed to conceal throughout her journey to China. She gave it to a cleaner at the camp in exchange for a bottle of fortified alcohol, which burned her mouth as she forced herself to gulp it down. She passed out.

The next thing she remembered was waking up in a military hospital where doctors had pumped her stomach. The experience left her with digestive problems for the rest of her life.

"I was in a room on my own, and they came in one by one. They barely even looked at you, they weren't bothered when we were in pain," she told me of her experiences. "And as soon as they finished, it was time for the next one." She lived for eight years like this, until the age of twenty-two.

After Guangdong, she was transported to Hong Kong and other bases around the Pacific. She ended up in Singapore, where, after its liberation by American and British troops, she was set free and was able to finally board a ship to return home.

In front of her family, she kept up the pretense that she had worked in a factory, daring not to share the truth. Only when her mother became insistent with her, following repeated refusals to get married, did she find the courage to tell her. Her mother died afterward of a heart attack that Kim believed was linked to her distress.

She never married and never spoke to anyone else about her war experience. She was lonely. She drank and smoked heavily. Not until she was in her sixties, four decades later, did she finally break her silence, inspired by women's rights groups in South Korea that had begun campaigning.

It took until 1991, forty-six years after the official end of World War II, for the first "comfort women" to speak out in public in Korea. The woman who broke the silence, Kim Hak-sun, decided to testify in public because of the fury she felt and the uncontrollable crying fits she experienced every time she heard the Japanese government deny that the sexual slavery system existed.

Her decision to come forward and then launch a legal claim against Japan spurred dozens of other women from Korea, the Philippines, China, Australia, and the Netherlands to tell their own stories. It was like a #MeToo moment of the pre-internet age, with each new testimony convincing others to step forward. In all, there were more than two hundred women, a tiny fraction of the total number.

Kim Bok-dong was among them. She spoke out in 1992. The same year, she joined protests that were taking place every Wednesday at noon in front of the Japanese embassy in Seoul to demand a full formal apology and compensation.

The protests continue to this day with the children and grandchildren of survivors sustaining the campaign. They hold banners and yellow butterflies, a symbol of freedom from violence. Opposite the embassy is a statue in bronze of a young girl dressed in traditional Korean clothing, sitting alone and upright in a chair, her fists clenched with determination. Her stare falls impassively on the diplomatic compound. Next to her is an empty chair inviting others to sit in her shoes.

"We want them to recognize that we were victims," Kim told me softly, looking up from behind her glasses. "I know that I am only staying alive to hear their apology. I want to hear it on behalf of all the others who have died before me."

More than twenty-five years after going public, she said she felt tired of having to continue to campaign, to talk about the rapes to journalists and audiences. She never expected the fight would take so long.

In 1993, following a first investigation, the chief cabinet secretary of the Japanese government at the time issued a written statement acknowledging that "comfort stations" existed and expressing "sincere apologies and remorse." But this was dismissed as insufficient by Kim and others who continued to press for an official apology from the state and compensation.

Even now, some politicians on Japan's nationalist Right insist the women were willing prostitutes. In 2007, more than forty parliamentarians paid for a full-page advertisement in *The Washington Post* falsely claiming that "no historical document has ever been found" showing that women were forced into prostitution against their will. In 2014, the Japanese government conducted a review of the original apology, reopening the wounds of the surviving grandmothers.

The issue is still not settled, partly because of the action of South Korea's former president Park Geun-hye, who has since been jailed for bribery and abuse of power. She negotiated what was called a "final and irreversible" settlement with the Japanese government in 2015, under which Tokyo agreed to apologize and pay one billion yen (around $10 million at the time) to a foundation to support survivors. In return, Japan demanded the removal of the statue in front of its embassy in Seoul.

But even though the agreement was in their name, none of the survivors had been consulted by President Park. They felt betrayed and overlooked in the name of patching up diplomatic relations. They refused the deal, which was frozen by Park's successor.

In January 2019, five months after I met her, Grandma Kim passed away in Seoul. She had been suffering from cancer during my visit. She held on to the dream of receiving a full apology to her dying breath and had wanted to spend any compensation money she received on a fund for schooling girls, having missed out on a large part of her own education. Her final words were an expression of disgust at her treatment.

It is not only Japan that has struggled to come to terms with the legacy and responsibility of its wartime actions. The victors in World War II have their own blind spots.

In 2014, Russian president Vladimir Putin signed a law into force that criminalizes "spreading false information about the activity of the USSR during the years of World War Two," making it now dangerous to even raise the mass rapes conducted by Red Army soldiers in Germany, which are officially denied.

The history of sexual violence committed by Allied forces in defeated Japan—Americans, British, Australian, and Indian troops as part of the British Commonwealth Occupation Force—remains another little-known chapter of the war. In just over a week between August 30 and September 10, 1945, 1,336 rapes by Allied forces were committed in a single province, Kanagawa, which lies to the south of Tokyo.[3]

Gripped by fear, the Japanese government set up a nationwide brothel system known as the "Recreation and Amusement Association," forcing prostitutes and other trafficked women to "service" foreign troops. Though using prostitutes was officially banned for Allied forces, commanders turned a blind eye.

In France, the Office of the Judge Advocate General for the European Theater of Operations concluded that "the number of violent sex crimes enormously increased with the arrival of our troops in France" after the Allied landing in Normandy in 1944.

My point is not that all soldiers are rapists or that we should stop paying tribute to the sacrifices and acts of bravery that they make during armed conflicts. This would be absurd and wrong. But we need to remember that there are valorous soldiers and predatory ones. And assaulted women deserve to be remembered, looked after, and compensated just as much as injured veterans or prisoners of war. Their injuries might not be visible, but they can last a lifetime.

There are fewer than two dozen grandmothers in Korea who are still alive to carry the flame of their movement. Grandma Kim's work was not in vain, however bitter and disillusioned she might have felt at the end of her life. At least ten statues and memorials dedicated to "comfort women" have been installed in the United States, often despite official objections from Japan. There are other public tributes in Vietnam and the Philippines.

The spirit of Grandma Kim lives on in the weekly protests, in these memorials, in the moving 2019 documentary *My Name Is Kim Bok Dong,* and in the annual prize named in her honor that recognizes other women who are following in her footsteps.

The recipient in 2019 was Vasfije Krasniqi-Goodman, a remarkable woman who leads a women's rights group in Kosovo and is a forceful member of SEMA, our global network of survivors of wartime sexual violence. In 1999, Vasfije was sixteen years old, the youngest daughter of a large family caught up in a war that saw Kosovo, with its population of mostly Muslim and ethnic Albanians, break away from Christian, Serb-dominated Yugoslavia.

One day, a Serbian policeman came to her family home, looking for her father and brother. They were away, but the policeman insisted she accompany him, ripping her from her mother's arms and threatening to shoot other relatives who tried to intervene.

She was targeted simply because she was Muslim. The policeman, who had a bandage on one of his hands, had been shot recently by ethnic Albanian forces. Both he and another older man raped her.

It took Vasfije nineteen years to speak out. When she did, she became the first Kosovar woman to accuse her attackers publicly. She has since become an advocate for the estimated twenty thousand women who suffered the same fate, most of whom continue to suffer in silence, feeling ashamed or fearful of the stigma they will encounter.

The policeman and the old man who raped Vasfije have escaped punishment, however, as is so often the case. Despite eyewitness testimony from her family about her abduction, the Kosovo Supreme Court overturned their guilty findings in a lower court on a legal technicality in 2014. No one has been convicted for rapes committed during the war in Kosovo or Serbia.

But Vasfije turned her anger and disappointment into the energy that drives her campaigning. She addressed the UN Human Rights Council, the US House of Representatives, and a host of conferences on behalf of other survivors. She is now an elected member of Kosovo's parliament focused on women's rights.

And thanks to lobbying from women's groups, and vocal support from the country's female president, Atifete Jahjaga, Kosovo has a pioneering compensation fund for survivors. It offers a lifetime monthly compensation of up to \$275—about 90 percent of the average salary for Kosovar women. The process is bureaucratic and requires women to prove their eligibility, which can be frustrating and provoke a second wave of traumatization. I met several despairing survivors who had had their applications refused.

But the program represents real progress: it is public recognition of the damage done by rape, of the existence of survivors, of their need to be remembered and looked after alongside soldiers wounded during the fighting. It also helps the healing process, compensating partly for the failures of the justice system to prosecute the perpetrators.

Despite its highly patriarchal culture, Kosovo is fighting back against stigma and helping survivors in other ways, too. In the center of the capital, Pristina, stands a five-meter-high monument called *Heroinat* (*Heroines*). It is made of twenty thousand metal pins, all capped with military-style medals featuring a woman's face, one for each rape victim during the war. I laid flowers there when I visited in late 2019 and was pleased to see how it had become a tourist attraction.

It is perhaps a sign of progress, the silver lining found in the succession of wars that continue to disfigure our planet, that survivors of sexual violence appear to be finding it easier to come forward and demand recognition for themselves and others.

Grandma Kim and her fellow Korean taboo smashers took more than four decades to come forward and speak about their experiences after World War II. Vasfije took nineteen years to defy the smothering silence that surrounded the rapes of the war in Kosovo. But when the Islamic State group created its system of sexual slavery of Yazidi women starting in 2014, women came forward almost immediately after they had escaped their captors, speaking to journalists and informing the world from refugee camps in northern Iraq.

The most remarkable among them was Nadia Murad, who became the face of the suffering of Yazidi women. Within a year, she had been invited to address the UN Security Council in New York by Samantha Power, the United States' UN ambassador. The speed with which she was recognized was a sign that our institutional mechanisms to identify and condemn mass sexual violence are improving.

Nadia told the UN how her six brothers had been shot by ISIS fighters, how she had been sold, humiliated, raped, and beaten. She delivered every word with such force, her trembling hands a sign of the difficulty of delivering such personal revelations to a room of strangers in unfamiliar surroundings. When she had finished, the room of normally impassive diplomats broke into applause.

Again and again, like Grandma Kim, she summoned up in public and to journalists the painful memories of her peaceful family life in Iraq before the war, the slaying of her brothers and relatives, and intimate details about her experiences at the hands of ISIS fighters. We should never forget the sacrifices made by women such as Nadia, Vasfije, Grandma Kim, or Tatiana Mukanire, Bernadette, and Jeanne, my cherished former patients in Congo, who speak out on behalf of others.

In 2018, the Nobel committee recognized Nadia's heroic campaigning work by awarding her the Nobel Peace Prize, naming me as her co-recipient. The award provided both of us with the biggest platform we'd ever had to speak out about sexual violence. It should be seen as part of the encouraging trend of recognizing the importance of the issue, even if it continues to occur with almost complete impunity in conflict zones now from Congo to Libya, Syria, Myanmar, or Nigeria.

I was in Bukavu when the Nobel committee made its announcement. It was a Friday, and at the time I was in the theater, operating on a perineum, surrounded by colleagues going about their work with their usual quiet concentration and professionalism. As we were finishing, we became aware of a commotion outside the building.

My first thought was that there was perhaps a fire or a security problem. But the shouts grew clearer and I could hear cheering and then ululating. Our anesthetist left the room to investigate as I was completing the last stitches. She returned moments later and flung her arm around my neck and hugged me.

"Papa, you've won the Nobel Prize!" she shouted.

I was stunned as each member of the team congratulated me. I finished my work with the patient and stumbled out of the operating theater in my gown and face mask. In the corridor outside, I could hear the crowd. At the entrance to the surgical bloc, dozens of patients from our survivors' wing had gathered along with staff.

I went outside to greet them, blinking in the sunlight. They cheered and broke into song. I was trying to make sense of the news as I felt arms around me and movement. It reminded me of how we had all danced together with V when she had visited the hospital for the first time back in 2007.

Back then it was a release from tension. This time it was a celebration of something that surpassed my personal achievement. It represented something much bigger. It was a celebration of the fact that the world seemed to be finally paying attention to the women of Congo. After two decades of feeling overlooked, being treated as insignificant, this was recognition that my patients' lives mattered.

So often over the years, survivors have stepped forward to speak to foreign journalists, UN officials, and diplomats in Bukavu, confiding in them their devastating personal stories in order to inform the world about what was happening. Afterward, they would often feel despondent, seeing that nothing seemed to change. I would try to reassure them, telling them that every contribution made a difference.

The Nobel Prize was recognition that their work and sacrifice had not been in vain.

The crowd grew bigger and bigger as cars and motorbikes blew their horns on the road outside the hospital. I made my way slowly toward my office, taking in the faces filled with joy in a place that has known so many tears. I walked past the consulting rooms where thousands of wretched stories have tumbled out over the years; past the metal entrance gate and its menacing razor wire, which I have always wished we could do without; past the blooming rows of red and pink roses that lift me every morning when I arrive for work.

I reached my office and thanked everyone who had accompanied me along the way. I walked in and closed the door, slumping into my trusty brown armchair. I felt happy, delighted, a touch delirious, proud, surprised, overwhelmed. It was a kaleidoscope of emotions.

Two conclusions emerged quickly: I was humbled to share the award with Nadia, whom I had already met several times. And I knew it would mean something and serve a purpose only insofar as it helped bring an end to the misery in Congo that had led to my nomination in the first place.

I've received various prizes over the years and I've tried to use each one as a platform to further the ideas you have read about in this book. On every occasion, the public recognition has made me feel hopeful, which has usually been followed by disillusionment with the ever-worsening living conditions in eastern Congo and the seemingly endless violence.

Over the following two months, I worked on my speech for the acceptance ceremony, which was held in Oslo in December. How should I use the opportunity of addressing royalty and politicians as well as a television audience of millions? I wrote and rewrote at night, or in the early hours of the morning, when I find

I am at my freshest, free from the demands of staff, patients, and visitors.

The challenges were much the same as for writing this book. I felt I needed to be explicit about the suffering I had witnessed, without searching to deliberately shock. I wanted to force listeners to think, without being overly provocative. Above all, I wanted to remind everyone of our collective responsibility for the disaster in Congo, not just as consumers of products that depend on minerals mined there but as fellow humans, members of a family that bleeds and suffers in the same way everywhere.

I've never watched a tape of my address. I've never been able to bear seeing myself in recordings or on television. I had memorized almost all of my speech during hours of practicing, and it all flashed by in an instant. I remember the sound of my voice reverberating in the huge, cavernous reception room of Oslo City Hall where the ceremony is held every year.

There were no nasty shocks like the sight of the empty chairs of the Congolese delegation at the UN in 2006. I could see Madeleine in the front row and my children among the two blocs of impeccably dressed guests in evening wear.

I spoke about the attack on my hospital in Lemera, the bloody start to our work at Panzi, our horror at the stream of children arriving from Kavumu. I reminded everyone of the millions of deaths and hundreds of thousands of rapes over twenty years. I stressed how the phones in everyone's pockets and the dazzling jewelry on display were part of the problem.

I brought up the UN Mapping Report that cataloged war crimes and crimes against humanity and was now "gathering mold in an office drawer in New York." I'd hoped this might spark fresh interest, that journalists might take a fresh look at its contents and begin questioning the lack of action.

I'm not sure how many people watched it back home. It was shown live by a host of international broadcasters, but not by state television in Congo, the only national channel in my country. They programmed a basketball game instead.

The most important consequence of the prize was that it afforded me an opportunity to expand my work. Immediately afterward, I began lobbying for an idea we had proposed after our fact-finding mission in Shabunda nearly ten years earlier when we had gone to interview survivors.

I'd never forgotten the women who spoke to us about their desire for recognition and the different forms it could take: schools for their children, money to start businesses or to buy land, funds for psychological care and health facilities, and public recognition. Our report at the end, submitted to the Office of the UN High Commissioner for Human Rights, had suggested setting up an international fund for survivors, funded by donors, that would try to meet some of these demands.

The idea never got off the ground. The only foreign government to take up the initiative was Brazil, whose president at the time, Dilma Rousseff—a woman—pledged $1 million. That was the end of it. No other government responded.

After the Nobel award and in the supportive environment created by the #MeToo movement, I felt I had an opportunity to rekindle the idea. Germany under Chancellor Angela Merkel agreed to sponsor a proposition for a global fund for survivors of sexual violence at the UN Security Council. It was approved by world powers in April 2019 as part of Resolution 2467.

Six months later, Nadia and I launched it publicly. France immediately came forward with a pledge of more than $6 million and the European Union a further $2 million. Japan has made a contribution of several million dollars, while the United Kingdom and South Korea have also agreed to provide financing. I am still hopeful that the United States will one day join in.

Our first projects are in Guinea in West Africa, Congo, and Iraq. The fund does many things, always with the aim of recognizing and compensating survivors. The guiding philosophy is that it will always be run and led by survivors, for other survivors. It will ask what they require and respond accordingly.

Part of the work is financing groups to make sure survivors can organize and their voices are heard. It will also offer technical advice to governments looking to set up compensation schemes of the sort I described in Kosovo. There are so many women around the world who find themselves in a lonely battle to recover, overlooked or deliberately neglected by their governments.

Take the Rohingya women who have been driven from their homes in Myanmar by a campaign of anti-Muslim killing and mass rape by government forces. They are massed in filthy refugee camps in neighboring Bangladesh. Who will provide the specialist care they require or do the vital lobbying work to highlight their needs?

In 2019, I traveled to Nigeria to meet some of the victims of Boko Haram, the Islamic extremist group active in the north of the country that has targeted women and girls. In 2014, they were responsible for abducting nearly three hundred schoolgirls in the village of Chibok, sparking the social media campaign known as #BringBackOurGirls.

About two hundred of their captives have since been released, but one hundred remain unaccounted for in 2021. I met a few of the survivors at a conference where they stood up and spoke about their needs. Some of the Chibok girls received government scholarships after they were released and even offers to study in the United States thanks to the campaign for them. But there are hundreds of other girls affected by the conflict whose schooling has been disrupted.

There is little hope for justice for them and scant financial support. The biggest desire of the girls I heard from was for education. Our fund and my foundation are looking into ways that we can help.

This is why the Nobel Peace Prize meant so much to me. It was recognition for the tens of thousands of women who have passed through our hospital in Bukavu. It sent a message that they matter. It gave me a platform to speak out about the Congo conflict, the search for justice, and the need for world powers to use their influence to tackle the cause of the fighting. But beyond the gesture and the speeches, it is being turned into action.

The check I received for $500,000 has been put to good use. The money has been used to buy property in the Congolese capital, Kinshasa, where we are opening a new facility for survivors, putting everything that we have learned in Bukavu at the service of a new and unserved population.

The women of Shabunda remain an inspiration. I hope we will one day have other statues like theirs across the country recognizing the resilience of the survivors who bear the scars of this unlamented period when Congo was labeled the rape capital of the world. I can still picture the agonized figure of the woman cast in bronze on her haunches. Public recognition like this helps lift survivors back to their feet.

The work of acknowledging and remembering survivors is part of the battle, components of the collective response that includes speaking out about sexual violence publicly and improving the criminal justice system. But all of these essential tasks, the focus of the last three chapters, are remedies to the problem. Like my time in the hospital's operating theater, they are dealing with the consequences of sexual violence once it has already happened, not the causes. Women should not need lifting back to their feet.

To prevent rapes from happening, we must ask ourselves why there are so many badly educated and poorly behaved men in the world in the first place—and why good, respectful men have stayed silent for so long.

9

MEN AND MASCULINITY

$\mathcal{M}$y reflections on men and masculinity must start with a basic personal question about my self-identity: Why am I the man I am? I do not intend to hold myself up as a role model. I have plenty of faults, as my wife, Madeleine, can attest to. I was not brought up as a male feminist, a concept neither of my parents, nor I, would have understood. Yet my education as a boy was different from that of others, and this clearly influenced the man I became, the professional choices I made, and my attitudes toward women.

I was raised in a household that challenged some but not all of the rigid ideas about gender roles that predominate in all patriarchal societies, not just in African ones. I was the third child born to my parents, after two sisters, and under Congolese tradition, I became the heir to the family.

The birth of the first boy in any Congolese family is a cause for celebration. Not only does it ensure the continuation of the family line—guaranteeing that the name will be passed down to the children of the subsequent generation—but it has important financial implications. Only boys inherit property and other assets from their fathers. As a consequence, boys are put on a pedestal from the moment they are born, which they grow more and more aware of as they mature.

One of the ways this becomes apparent in Congolese families, still today, is that boys are exempted from housework and are not required to take part in the daily tasks of domestic life. Their sisters are expected to clean, cook, and wash once they are old enough. Worse, they are then expected to attend to the boys, creating a clear hierarchy understandable to even the greenest of young minds.

Except at home with the Mukweges.

For reasons that are unclear, my mother had rather progressive views about the roles and responsibilities of her children. I suspect it was mostly because of her difficult and precarious childhood, owing to the death of her mother and the rejection she experienced from her father. She was unusually reliant on a male figure as a caregiver—her older brother, who went out daily in search of food and watched over her and her two sisters.

Her brother demonstrated that men, too, could handle domestic work that was normally reserved for women. And having experienced the need to fend for themselves at such a young age, my mother wanted to transmit the skills that had enabled her and her siblings to survive. She wanted us to be self-sufficient. "You need to be able to look after yourself without depending on anyone," she used to tell us.

As a result, she forced me to do "girl's work" such as washing up or the laundry as soon as I was old enough. She obliged me to make my bed and clean my own shoes before leaving for school, jobs that my sisters would have traditionally been expected to do.

At first, I resisted and found my mother unfair and unnecessarily strict. I remember going to friends' houses and seeing how their sisters waited on them. As soon as we finished eating, we would return to our games or homework while the girls cleared up. As a young boy, I craved the same privileges.

But gradually I took to the work and eventually enjoyed the sensation of self-reliance and contributing. It became awkward around the age of twelve and in my early adolescence when friends would come to our house. "Why are you doing girl's stuff?" they'd ask. My older sisters' friends were equally bemused. They saw me as a curiosity and would giggle and make jokes as I did the laundry or ironing.

But all those skills came in handy when I lived alone as a young adult in Kinshasa, Bujumbura, and France. And I believe my mother's egalitarian approach had a profound impact on how I saw women. From my first memories, I was not encouraged to believe that I was superior to my sisters or exempt from the chores of life. On the contrary, my older sister Elizabeth was held in great esteem by my parents, particularly my father, which rubbed off on me. How can we expect men to respect women and treat them as equals if they are given power over their submissive sisters from their earliest memories?

I developed an extremely close relationship with my sister Roda, who is two years older than me. We were partners and accomplices in work and in play. She was the biggest beneficiary of my first ventures into the business world as a teenager, when I would sell fizzy drinks from the bottom of our garden. With my earnings, I'd buy her dresses and shoes. When she put them on, I was filled with pride. At other times, I'd help her out, doing jobs around the house to make her happy. We were a team.

But this is not how most boys grow up. They become aware of their gender-determined privileges at a young age through their treatment at home and their relationships with their sisters or other girls their age. In fact, the discrimination starts even earlier than this. It begins in most countries even before children have been born.

At the hospital, when I have pregnant patients for their consultation who have had one or two daughters already, they are always desperate to find out the sex of their next child. On so many occasions I have had to console them when I break the news that they are carrying another daughter. A few years ago, I stopped informing my patients about the gender of their babies for this reason.

I understand the importance they attach to boys. They live in a system that places value on male heirs. Their status depends on giving birth to sons.

Through tears after an ultrasound scan, many have confided in me how they fear returning home because their husbands may beat them for having another girl. Some, who have had three or four girls in a row, know that they risk being divorced or forced into polygamy, which is illegal but still practiced. It is still socially acceptable in some communities for the husband to take another wife if his first one delivers too many girls.

This deeply rooted gender preference explains why such catastrophic imbalances have been recorded in some areas of India and China in particular. In both places, female feticide—the selective abortion of female fetuses—has led to populations heavily skewed toward men. It's clearly seen in their birth rates, showing that 106 to 108 boys are born for every 100 girls in both countries.[1] There are millions of "extra" men and "missing" women, causing a host of documented social problems including "bride-napping" and higher levels of violence.

The gender hierarchy is spelled out and reinforced in thousands of other ways throughout the life of a girl and boy, from their earliest memories into adolescence and then adulthood. It takes place from the womb to the grave. The message is always the same: that a male life is superior to a female one.

When my father died, I and my brothers inherited his estate, not my sisters. As the oldest boy, I symbolically took over as head of the family at that time in a ceremony that takes place at the end of the funeral service.

It is led by a maternal uncle—a holdover from the matriarchal customs of the precolonial era—who, under tradition, hands over the family's weapons, such as a machete or a spear, to the oldest son. He might also hand over copper bracelets or hunting prizes such as leopard skins or teeth, which were seen as signs of strength and bravery. In the modern era, the uncle usually bestows symbolic possessions such as a suit jacket or watch.

My uncle gave me my father's most cherished Bible, his first one, which had yellowed and well-worn pages. It contained notes in pencil, as well as the date he had first read each passage. I also received his cane, which he had used during his long walks as a traveling evangelist in the 1940s. Sadly, the Bible was lost during a trip to Paris some years ago when my bag was stolen at the airport's luggage carousel.

At the end of the funeral ceremony, my siblings were invited to pay their respects. Under Congolese paternalistic tradition, they recognized me from then on as the head of the family, even referring to me as "papa." I am expected to look out for them and manage the family's estate. It was a far cry from the days of doing the dishes with my sisters.

None of us can escape tradition, and neither should we feel we have to. The customs and ceremonies of life form the grammar of our existence and are important in nurturing our identities and sense of self. But it is important to question them. We must open our eyes to their impact. Whenever we reinforce the message that boys are more capable, more deserving, or more valuable, we perpetuate injustice—and ultimately violence—against women.

Why do I say violence? What is the link between the division of domestic chores, inheritance traditions, or funeral ceremonies and rape? It is that the more boys and men are made to believe they are superior, that their lives matter more, the more likely they are to conclude that they have a right to dominate and mistreat other people's daughters and sisters physically.

It is not just fathers who entrench gender biases in children. Mothers, too, are responsible. I've often wondered if mothers pamper their boys, raising them like princes and taking such pride in their physical strength and virility, because they live vicariously through them. They educate their sons to take up all the privileges and advantages that have been denied to them. It's a sort of payback for all the indignities suffered during their lifetime of submission. This is part of the challenge we face.

Changing centuries of cultural conditioning is difficult, but most countries are making progress in tackling some of the crushing institutionalized biases against women that have built up like sediment over centuries, owing to laws created and enforced by self-serving men.

In 2019, I had the privilege of co-presiding over a working group on women's rights for the G-7 summit hosted by French president Emmanuel Macron, who put gender equality at the heart of the official agenda. The meeting in the town of Biarritz brought together the leaders of the world's richest democracies: the United States, Canada, the United Kingdom, France, Germany, Italy, and Japan.

During our work, we looked at the unequal treatment of women and girls around the globe and concluded that 2.5 billion of them—almost half—lived in countries with laws that discriminated against them. It took a variety of forms: in some countries, women are still unable to inherit property, or do commercial work, or take a job without their husbands' permission. Some legislation prevents them from opening bank accounts on their own or taking out a loan to start a business. There are multiple examples of discriminatory divorce, citizenship, and child custody laws.

We produced a list of seventy-nine examples of gender-neutral laws that could serve as inspiration for countries to tackle violence against women, improve economic empowerment, and reduce discrimination in education and health. It's surprising how much work remains to be done, even in countries that see themselves as women-friendly. For example, around 80 percent of Americans believe that the US Constitution explicitly guarantees equal rights to men and women. In fact, they're mistaken.

The Founding Fathers made no explicit reference to men and women being equal Americans. Women are seen as being covered by the Fourteenth Amendment in the part of its first section known as the Equal Protection Clause, which was passed in 1868 in order to extend equal rights and protection to freed (male) slaves. It has since been interpreted by the US Supreme Court as extending civil rights to all Americans, including women. This is not the same thing as stating explicitly that men and women are equals.

To rectify this historic oversight, the US Congress passed what is known as the Equal Rights Amendment (ERA) in 1972, which would have added to the Constitution that "equality of rights under the law shall not be denied or abridged by the United States or by any state on account of sex."

It was sent for ratification by US states, and thirty-five of them promptly approved it—three short of the thirty-eight needed for the amendment to pass. As the process neared its end, the legislation became bogged down in a fierce culture war over the role of women in society and abortion rights. Momentum stalled and it never made it onto the statute book.

In recent years, Nevada, Illinois, and Virginia have ratified, thanks to an uptick in interest following the #MeToo campaign, but a legal challenge from the Trump administration and opposition in the Republican-controlled Senate prevented it from passing into law in 2020. Groups such as the ERA Coalition, cofounded by my friend Jessica Neuwirth, continue campaigning for it to be completed in what would amount to a major symbolic victory, a century after women were first given the right to vote.

And symbolism matters. As individuals, we are constantly absorbing signals about our place and status in society. They are often subtle and almost imperceptible, contained in language and our behavior, but they reinforce the damaging hierarchy of gender—and race, of course, which the Black Lives Matter movement has brought to the fore.

But even when legislation is passed guaranteeing women equal treatment, the lag between changing laws and changing attitudes is often a process that takes place over decades. One need only look at the gender pay gap in Western countries to see the gap between lawmaking and progress. After half a century of regulatory action designed to root out discrimination in the home, schools, and workplace, the salaries of men and women are still starkly different when they perform the same tasks.

The latest figures from the OECD show that full-time working men were paid on average 13 percent more than women across thirty-six of its member countries, but this headline figure hides major discrepancies.[2] The gap was around 18 percent in the United States and Canada, 24 percent in Japan, and 16 percent in the United Kingdom. The earnings of the part-time employed and self-employed show a much larger shortfall for women across all countries. Women company owners in the United States, for example, earn around half as much as their male counterparts. The shortfall for people of color is even larger.

Statistics for the gap in income—which measures all forms of income, not just wages—on a global basis between men and women paint an even starker picture of the biases. The World Economic Forum, which has been tracking the global gender gap since 2004, estimates that men have almost double the annual income of women, at $21,000 versus $11,000 at purchasing power parity, an economic measure that accounts for currency differences. And while the wage gap might be falling at a slow rate in Western democracies, it is actually growing in the rest of the world.[3]

Wage gaps, discriminatory laws, male-dominated social conventions, the unfair division of domestic work, and the underrepresentation of women in positions of authority, which I will elaborate on later, all underline the corrosive message that women's lives are not as valuable as men's.

We run several community programs aimed at correcting biases against women and girls in Congo. While nondiscriminatory laws are important, the grassroots work of civil society groups is essential. Often communities and individuals need help, a nudge and some gentle persuasion, in order to question their behavior or experience the benefits for themselves. Such work is laborious and time-consuming. It requires energy and investment over long time periods. I have seen the results with my own eyes, but I have also been confronted with the difficulties.

I want to tell you a story that was important in helping me understand the complexity of the issue and the challenge we face in encouraging parents to value their girls as much as boys. It underscored to me why we cannot simply condemn or judge parents when they raise their sons as princes and treat their daughters like slaves. They are often reacting to the customs and traditions that shape their lives.

Our foundation in Panzi has a program to encourage girls to attend school in the area. As I explained in previous chapters, we operate in a poor district of Bukavu, made up of a warren of mud roads and lanes lined with shacks and huts. The schools, like everywhere else in Congo, are run by church organizations and are private.

The poorest parents often cannot afford to educate all of their offspring. The average number of children per family in Congo is around six, and the most vulnerable tend to have larger families than the more educated and wealthier ones. A big family is seen as long-term security, and for the poorest among us, children are the only reliable and free source of joy.

School fees therefore account for a large part of household expenditure for most families in Panzi, as they were for my family when I was growing up. With limited resources, many parents prioritize sending boys to school over girls as a result.

We wanted to reach some of the poorest girls around Panzi who were not being given an opportunity to learn. The foundation set up a program in which parents could enroll their daughters and we would cover the fees and provide an education kit comprising all the basics, such as a bag, pencils, pens, and paper.

In 2015, I attended a ceremony to meet some of the parents who were benefiting from the program. Looking through the list of parents and their children beforehand, I noticed that there were a surprisingly large number of pupils enrolled who had gender-neutral first names. They were supposed to be girls, but they could also have been boys. It was impossible to tell.

My interest was piqued. Making sure our money is properly targeted in a country of endemic fraud requires constant attention.

After the formalities of the ceremony, I began talking to the parents. Most of them were laborers and vendors from the Panzi area, the sorts of people who can be seen sitting at roadside stalls for twelve hours a day or pushing carts and toiling on construction sites. Most had brought their children.

I began chatting with a mother who was on her own. She told me her daughter was called Bahati—one of the gender-neutral names that cropped up on the enrollment lists. I asked after her. "Where is she? I'd like to meet her," I said.

She hadn't been able to come, the mother explained. I sensed unease and embarrassment. I pressed a bit more. "Who is she with? Could you call her to come? It's important that all the children meet the people from the foundation," I said.

Unable to answer, she stared down at the floor. Then, without looking up, she told me her story.

She was a widow, and she sold bananas in the street in front of the hospital. It was long, tiring work, sitting by the road in the traffic fumes and noise of impatient drivers blowing their horns. It earned her less than a dollar a day. This meant she didn't make enough to be able to educate all of her children. When she heard about the foundation's work, she saw an opportunity. She signed up her son.

"If I send one of my girls, as soon as she finishes her studies, she'll get married and go to live with her husband's family and help them," she said. "She won't stay with me. What's the use?"

She was wrongly claiming aid money intended for marginalized girls. But I felt sympathy for her. She faced a daily battle with hunger, illness, and the physical discomfort of extreme poverty, as well as the guilt of knowing she was failing to provide adequately for all her children.

And what she described was true. We live in a society in which girls are property passed from one family to another at the time of marriage, when the bride swaps her father's surname for her husband's. This woman's daughter, unless she succeeded so well at school that she could pursue a career and defy her low social status, would in all probability be married in her late teens and leave her mother for good. It didn't justify the woman's actions, but it explained them.

Our education program continues, with regular checks on the children who receive assistance. We spend hundreds of thousands of dollars a year in this way, helping between three thousand and five thousand children annually.

Our challenge as a society is convincing parents to believe in their daughters' abilities. As has happened in the West over several decades, the more opportunities there are for women to fulfill their potential and find roles for themselves outside the home, the more parents will invest in their education.

I remember a conversation with a man who was receiving kidney dialysis at the hospital a few years ago. I walked past him in a waiting room and he jumped to his feet to thank me for the help his family had received. He gripped my hand very tightly as he said how touched he was that as a Muslim he had not been discriminated against.

Had the foundation not offered to pay the school fees for his daughter, he confessed, he would not have invested in her education. She was destined for marriage and child-rearing. The man had several sons who were his priority.

But nothing had worked out how he imagined. His daughter had studied hard, earned her high school diploma, and found an accounting job at a local company. She was married, but her wages gave her financial independence. His boys had proved less successful.

"She's the one paying for my treatment now," he explained. "I was wrong. Without her, I'd be dead."

For the last ten years, we have also been working with communities in eastern Congo aimed at promoting "positive masculinity" as part of our outreach program called Badilika ("Change"). It sees our volunteers travel to often remote villages to talk about human rights, holding the local government to account, and crucially the role of men and fathers who are heads of households.

In these rural communities, women always do the cooking and cleaning; they bear the children and serve as the primary caregivers. They cultivate crops to feed the family, doing the overwhelming majority of the backbreaking work of sowing, planting, and harvesting cassava, sweet potatoes, yams, beans, or corn. Once they are finished in the fields, they carry their production to market.

If the family cultivates cash crops such as coffee or nuts, men will sometimes deign to carry these. Cutting trees is also seen as a man's job, as is building and maintaining the home. Men hold the economic power through their management of the family purse, which they allocate to what they see as the household's priorities.

The responsibilities, and the energy required to accomplish their respective tasks, are vastly different. And to no one's surprise by now, I imagine, the biggest burden of work falls on women. It is common to see groups of men playing cards in villages while their wives are out in the fields or walking past, crippled by the weight of their loads. It is ludicrously unfair and infuriating to witness.

Yet the picture is more or less the same worldwide, evident in the many surveys of the amount of leisure time enjoyed by men and women, respectively. Men do far more paid work, but the burden of unpaid work—caring for children and elderly relatives, cleaning, shopping, and other household chores—falls overwhelmingly on women in heterosexual couples. In the thirty-seven leading democracies that are members of the OECD, women on average perform more than double the amount of unpaid work as men. And in every country, men have more time off.

The differences range from around thirty to forty minutes more leisure time per day for men in countries such as the United States, the United Kingdom, Australia, Germany, and Sweden, to around an hour more in France, India, and South Africa. Men have nearly an hour and a half extra in places such as Italy, Greece, and Portugal. Added up over a year, these differences amount to hundreds of hours of extra leisure time for men.

The novel coronavirus crisis served only to highlight these trends. With millions of couples all locked down together under the same roof, the discrepancy between the daily workload of men and women was clearer than ever. Marlène Schiappa, France's secretary of state for gender equality, spoke for many when she warned about the "silent exhaustion" of women as a result. The head of the International Monetary Fund, Kristalina Georgieva, warned in April 2021 about mothers with young children quitting their jobs, saying they were "among the biggest casualties of the economic lockdowns."

The problem is that men don't like being told they are macho.

They tend to be happy with their privileges, which free them from shouldering an equal burden of life's joyless tasks. Turning up in a village in Congo and lecturing the men about their games of rummy and blackjack while their wives are working is not going to change centuries of tradition.

In 2010, we began working with a tribe called the Warega, which hails from an area to the east of Bukavu. They number several million in total and have their own language, Kirega. Many have migrated to Bukavu over the years in search of work and security owing to the presence of armed groups across their territory.

We approached their tribal chiefs and spoke to them about the work we wanted to do, aimed at improving the status of women but also improving their farming practices. They were open to our ideas and, after traveling in person to the hospital for a first meeting, promised to support our outreach efforts.

These began with small voluntary seminars. We invited husbands and unmarried young men to attend meetings held in several villages in Warega communities. Those who accepted were more open-minded and disposed to change, of course, but they were all workingmen from traditional farming backgrounds.

The work started with a discussion about the role and responsibilities of women. The men were encouraged to evaluate all of the work done by their spouses. As they described their daily tasks, some expressed surprise, even mild embarrassment, as they totted up the long list of jobs their wives handled silently without complaint. Many admitted they almost never saw their wives relaxing.

Volunteers would write down all the tasks around a picture of a woman with half a dozen arms or more, rather like the Hindu deity Durga. But though Durga is usually depicted with hands holding weapons, the woman in our picture is doing cooking, cleaning, feeding, cultivating, and so on with hers.

Over a series of meetings, we would probe why some work was reserved for women and other tasks for men. This was how their parents had worked, and their grandparents before that, the men usually replied. Village life had always been this way.

The discussions would then move on to their personal finances. The educators would ask how much money they made from farming and whether there was enough food all year round. Families in the area generally struggled, and malnutrition was a major problem despite the incredibly rich soil. Looting from armed groups and the dangers of working out in the fields could be seen in the hollowed faces of many in the village.

The trainers—the teams are a mix of men and women—would also broach taboo issues such as menstruation, explaining the impact on women's bodies and energy levels, as well as the physical effects of pregnancy and the difficulty of working immediately before and after delivering children. We would also talk about the domestic chores for sons and daughters, as well as the attitudes toward educating girls.

At the end, the men were invited to identify jobs that they could help their wives with. The goal was to encourage them to think about ways in which they could team up with their wives to share some of the tasks. Some of the men worried about the reaction of others: if they were seen carrying their wives' crops, they might be laughed at for doing women's work.

The trainers stressed that by working together, they might be able to increase their farming yields. Or that by looking after the children more, they might free their wives to spend more time in the fields. They would be more efficient. And happier.

The suggestions were not embraced by everyone, perhaps only a minority initially. The process of changing culture often takes places over generations, because much of the time only young people are open to adopting new ideas. But we saw that several of the men were willing to try, particularly doing more farming together.

They ended up becoming the biggest advocates. Over several seasons, these early adopters returned and told others how they were able to produce more with their wives. The income enabled them to build more solidly. Some swapped their straw roofs for metal ones. Others confessed that their relationships with their wives and children were much better as a result of the changes they had made.

The results were so positive that the elders from the tribe invited me to visit their region, an invitation I was happy to accept. It provided an opportunity to deepen our work. The Badilika program has since been extended to three different regions and we work with fifteen different local Congolese partner organizations on a host of issues.

The methods vary from place to place. There are sometimes seminars, plays, or film projections that are aimed at sparking a discussion about the role and rights of women as well as sexual violence. Some of our partners run marriage workshops in which couples are invited to discuss their roles together. One group has shut down a local brothel complicit in recruiting girls. It's slow, community-level work, but real social change always takes place at this level.

The role of peer-to-peer transmission of the ideas in the Badilika program was absolutely crucial. There is only so much trainers and feminists can do on their own. Overall, we've found that men tend to be more receptive when the trainers are male, too. But the success of our work ultimately depends on a few early adopters in the community influencing others around them.

This brings me to the vital influence of male role models in changing attitudes toward women, and I want to return to my own childhood: I credit my mother with exposing me for the first time to the vital importance of equality at home in how she divided up the domestic chores between my sisters and me. But I must also acknowledge the influence of my father.

He was, and remains, an inspiration to me in many ways. I looked up to and admired him enormously as a boy for his commitment, wisdom, kindness, and generosity. Although he and my mother had a traditional relationship in many ways—I witnessed him cook only once, when my mother was very sick, and I never saw him clean—he was different from most men in one crucial aspect.

Papa was exceptional in that he never raised a hand or struck any of his children or my mother. His authority was unquestioned, however, and his ability to discipline was in no way impeded. I feared him pulling me aside for a conversation, and his look of deep disappointment at my behavior, far more than a thrashing.

I remember once climbing on the kitchen table and scribbling on the ceiling. I initially tried to blame my sister, an obvious lie that was soon exposed. That earned me a slap from my mother, but my father sat me down when he got home as usual at around five P.M. and delivered a lecture on the sanctity of our home and the importance of respect. I did my best to explain my behavior and murmured my apologies.

Researchers have found that exposure to domestic violence as a child—by either seeing their mother being struck or being struck themselves—is highly correlated with an individual's likelihood to commit violent acts as an adult.[4] This confirms what we know to be true from experience: that children copy their role models. To put it another way, fathers who beat their children or their wives are increasing the chances that their sons will in turn be violent with others later in life.

Domestic violence is extraordinarily widespread in Congo, as it is across most of Africa, parts of Asia, and the Middle East. A total of 57 percent of married Congolese women reported having experienced violence from their current or former husband, according to a 2014 survey from the Ministry of Health. Seventy-five percent of women agreed that it was acceptable for a husband or partner to beat his wife under certain circumstances, according to data from the OECD.

Domestic violence is still extremely prevalent, though less widespread, in developed countries. Even in Scandinavia, one in four women reported experiencing some form of intimate partner violence. The figures are the same for the larger European countries such as the United Kingdom, France, and Germany. In the United States, one in three women has been assaulted at least once.[5]

The home is an even more violent place for children. Between eight and nine out of ten children are subjected to violent discipline in Congo, according to data from UNICEF. The picture is much the same throughout Africa, the Middle East, and large parts of Asia.

Laws banning it have progressed over the last forty years when almost no states prohibited it entirely. Today there are fifty-eight states that make it illegal to hit children in any setting, including the home—most of Europe, South America, and eight African countries, including South Africa—but they represent just 12 percent of all minors globally, according to the Global Initiative to End All Corporal Punishment of Children.

The United States has no such legislation at the federal level and is the only major Western country where corporal punishment is still legal in some schools. A total of ninety-two thousand students were physically punished in 2015–2016, mostly in southern US states, according to the Department of Education's Office for Civil Rights.[6] Three-quarters of those beaten, slapped, or spanked were boys.

In the home, beatings are mostly carried out by fathers. Boys absorb the lesson that using force is somehow a characteristic of masculinity, an acceptable means of discipline and control. As adults, they resort to force or bullying when they encounter resistance or challenges.

As well as constantly reinforcing the message that their lives matter more, parents and society at large often explicitly reinforce the message to boys that being male and masculine is about strength and toughness: we encourage them not to cry; we make them believe that showing weakness or sensitivity is somehow "feminine"; we tell them not to show fear or be scared.

Studies have shown that parents react differently to the cries of children, even as babies, depending on whether they are male or female. The way we select toys, discipline, encourage, and love our children is often influenced by their gender.

Boys learn to bottle up their emotions as a consequence, leading to explosions of frustration when they're unable to express themselves with words.

I see the practical consequences of these lessons at the hospital, not just in the injuries sustained during fights between men but also on the bodies of battered wives and, of course, in the psychological and physical harm inflicted on victims of sexual violence. I also see it in the men who have put off consulting a doctor, giving illness and disease time to ravage their bodies, as if acknowledging they are sick is unmanly or weak. It is why prostate cancer is such a killer.

This macho conditioning of men to be fearless and brave also explains why they were less likely to wear a mask during the outbreak of COVID-19 in 2020, despite all the epidemiological evidence showing they were more likely to die.[7] Some politicians such as Donald Trump and Brazilian president Jair Bolsonaro made it a point of honor not to be seen wearing a face covering. Men were also less likely to wear masks during the SARS and H1N1 respiratory disease outbreaks in Asia, a separate study found.[8]

We as adults, parents, and caregivers are responsible for projecting these damaging male character traits onto children. I believe that "masculinity" is something that is acquired by children over the course of their lives. They are not born with it. It is a social construct. It's something a boy puts on like layers of clothing as he develops. The end result can be as varied as that statement implies.

The problem is that we force many children into a straitjacket of what men *should* be. We tell them there are masculine fashions they must adopt. The style is of someone who is strong, physical, dominating, who succeeds and subjugates. Resisting these rules is seen as weakness. And when boys adopt these male character traits too forcefully, we do not correct the excess.

When teenage boys turn into men, through a process of education and emulation, they have built up their masculine outerwear. It is often tough and brittle, something they find uncomfortable to carry but wrongly assume is superior.

When I look at the two major features of my upbringing—a mother who insisted on equality between my sisters and me at home and a nonviolent father—it helps me to understand why so many men grow up with an alternative, toxic understanding of their maleness. The lessons they absorb are exactly the opposite: they are told from birth that they are superior and that using physical force is acceptable and even necessary to gain respect.

It would be ridiculous to deny that there are differences between boys and girls—I have seen it with my own eyes with my children—but parents decide what traits to emphasize and curb depending on whether they see value in them. And we are all subject to centuries of gender conditioning, even the most open-minded among us.

We need to bring up boys without all the preconceived notions of manhood based on strength, power, and dominance. We need to give them freedom to express a full range of emotions, not suppress those considered "feminine" such as compassion, kindness, and sensitivity. We also need to talk to them a lot more about gender equality, gender roles, the importance of respecting women, and also—this is very important—about sex.

Men are said to be constantly thinking about sex, which makes it all the more puzzling to me that so many fathers are reluctant to talk about it with their sons. I don't mean joking about it or having lighthearted conversations about girls. I mean really talking about it.

In Congo, before a wedding, the bride will normally be taken aside by her female relatives, who will talk to her about her marriage night and answer any questions she might have about what may or may not be her first sexual experience. It's part of our culture, a rite of passage.

But nothing like this exists for grooms. It is just assumed that they know everything. And they never ask questions because that would be humiliating, an admission that they are ignorant about something they are simply expected to master.

I've observed it in Western countries, too. Mothers are generally comfortable talking to their daughters about sex at the appropriate age, seeing it as part of their responsibilities. Fathers will support this, being keen to protect their daughters, remembering their own behavior as teenagers and that of their peer group.

Beyond the practical advice given to girls, the conversations will also inevitably turn to the dangers of men and boys: the risk of falling pregnant and of being abused. The underlying message drilled into girls and women is always the same: "Don't get raped." We tell them to be careful about whom they meet, to avoid dangerous areas, to pay attention to what they wear, and to be cautious about the signals they send. They are urged to be on their guard and avoid making themselves vulnerable.

But much less time and attention are spent on the far more important lesson that should be directed again and again at boys. We need to be telling them: "Don't rape!" How many fathers sit down and actually talk to their sons about the nature of consent?

The father of Brock Turner, the college swimmer convicted for sexually assaulting an unconscious woman at Stanford University in 2016, became infamous after describing his son's behavior as "twenty minutes of action" that did not deserve a prison term. It's hard not to think that a twenty-minute conversation about consent before Brock went to the university could have avoided the whole disturbing saga.

In October 2015, the US sexual health-care charity Planned Parenthood funded a nationwide survey on consent. On every measure, such as whether foreplay could be considered consent for sex or whether a previous sexual encounter constituted consent for sex again, women were significantly better informed than men. It also showed that parents talked with their daughters more than their sons.[9]

And fathers shouldn't stop at talking about consent; they need to go further. There are so many things boys are ignorant about but are somehow assumed to know. What is good sex? Do they understand how prevalent sexual abuse is? We need to explain the fact that raping someone is never "twenty minutes of action" but may condemn someone to a lifetime of psychological pain. We need to tackle the tragic mismatch in perception of rape and its consequences between the perpetrators and the victims.

We need more well-informed boys to act as role models among their peers. Almost every man can think of situations where he was present when friends, teammates, or colleagues behaved inappropriately with women in front of him. We don't like to admit it, but these acts implicate us by association. Many men turn a blind eye; some may feel remorse afterward for failing to act. But we need a new generation of boys who will step in, be proactive, call out bad behavior, and influence their peers.

When Donald Trump made his infamous "grab 'em by the pussy" remark about women to *Access Hollywood* host Billy Bush while traveling with him and seven other men on a bus in 2005, he did not assume that Bush or the others approved of his methods necessarily. But he could count on no one being shocked. The laughter from his audience was testimony to this.

Bush, who was fired afterward, has spoken about his regret and shame for being complicit. During the height of the #MeToo movement, he wrote that the outpouring of stories about abuse were a "reckoning and reawakening, and I hope it reaches all the guys on the bus." Only by taking the sex education of our boys more seriously, not just in the home but in schools and universities, will this happen.

One disturbing new development of the last few decades is the impact of pornography, which is more prevalent and easily accessible than ever before. Setting aside the moral arguments about pornography, we should all be able to agree that the most popular sites host extreme and unhealthy content, showing degrading and often coercive acts perpetrated on generally submissive women.

Pornhub, the world's biggest open-access porn site, with forty-two billion visits in 2019, has profited from sexual abuse after videos of underage girls being raped were posted on its portal. It also hosted videos from an amateur porn production company since found to have tricked women into appearing in its videos.[10]

Defenders of pornography argue that it depicts sexual fantasies and serves as harmless erotica. Some researchers have suggested that pornography may actually help to reduce sexual violence, by offering masturbatory relief for would-be aggressors. But if we fail in our responsibility to educate boys about sex, there is clear evidence that they take their lessons from X-rated videos.

Young women today, who have grown up in the modern era of readily available internet pornography, are facing the consequences. Research done by the polling group Savanta ComRes for the BBC in November 2019 showed that more than a third of women in the

United Kingdom had experienced unwanted slapping, choking, gagging, or even spitting during consensual sex.

A meta-analysis published in December 2015 in the *Journal of Communication* by three US-based academics analyzed the effects of watching pornography based on the results of twenty-two studies from seven different countries.[11] Their conclusion was unequivocal: "The accumulated data leave little doubt that, on average, individuals who consume pornography more frequently are more likely to hold attitudes conducive to sexual aggression and engage in actual acts of sexual aggression than individuals who do not consume pornography or who consume pornography less frequently."

A more recent study in 2019 looking at US teens again showed a powerful link between exposure to violent pornography and dating violence. They found that male adolescents who were exposed to violent pornography were more than three times as likely to perpetrate sexual dating violence.[12]

The sheer quantity of pornography and the difficulty of restricting access to it make it more important than ever that we discuss it openly with our children, pointing out the various ways in which it depicts often unhealthy and unrealistic sexual experiences.

Most parents and schools consider it their responsibility to educate children in the basics of courtesy: how we should speak to each other and, in public, how to nurture healthy friendships. Yet we forget or neglect, often out of prudishness or embarrassment, to talk about sex. We leave that job to pornographers at our peril.

Positive role models—men who are prepared to call out toxic masculinity when they encounter it—are essential. It starts with fathers speaking to their sons in private, but we need many more public figures to join the struggle in a meaningful way. They must lead by example.

Sadly, the film, music, and video game industries continue to bombard young adults with depictions of men as muscular, aggressive, virile, and often misogynistic. The people who profit from these industries, and the stars who are followed by millions, must look at their own responsibilities. Campaign groups and activists can only keep up the pressure on them to mend their ways, calling out the worst examples of behavior that normalizes or promotes sexually aggressive conduct.

In 2008, two years after I met V for the first time in New York, she invited me to an event she was organizing in New Orleans to celebrate ten years of her V-Day organization. In her typical style, she wanted something bold, so she rented out the Superdome stadium, which was the scene of numerous sexual assaults after Hurricane Katrina, when it had been turned into a chaotic and squalid rescue center.

She renamed it the Superlove, and over the course of the weekend thirty thousand people came by to listen to talks, seek advice at healing and medical centers, and enjoy a performance of *The Vagina Monologues* starring Jane Fonda and Kerry Washington. Everyone walked into the stadium through an origami-style vulva that glowed in the dark.

V invited me to lead a march of hundreds of women through the city, ending at Congo Square, once known as Place des Negres, which had been the only area in the city where Black slaves were able to gather on Sundays in the late eighteenth and nineteenth centuries. But the main reason for my presence was to be given the first prize of a new organization she had created called V-Men, which brought together men working on women's rights.

The idea was to create a network of men who were not embarrassed to promote "women's issues." I had to walk out onstage through a curtain made of long threads of pink material hanging in the middle of two red cutouts in the shape of vaginal lips.

Naturally, most visitors to the Superlove were women, many of them women of color who had suffered disproportionately from the effects of Hurricane Katrina and the sexual violence that followed. During our panel discussion about V-Men afterward, which included the then Baltimore Ravens linebacker Bart Scott along with others, we wondered aloud what it would take to encourage more men to join us.

This is the next stage of the work that must take place following #MeToo. The cause of women's rights is not a cause for women alone. Men need to join in. They don't have to attend conferences or healing centers, still less be prepared to walk through a giant pink vagina onto a stage in public.

But they do need to speak up about sexual violence. They do need to embrace and act out alternative models of being a man, demonstrating that they can be strong and sensitive, brave and compassionate, resilient yet emotional, and everything in between. They do need to take more time to speak to their teenage sons, honestly and openly, about women's rights.

Never have there been as many men informed about and broadly sympathetic to the women's rights movement and the campaign to eliminate sexual violence as today. They need to take the next step, moving from being passive supporters to active participants in the social change we need. The responsibility for changing laws, demanding justice, denouncing abusers, working in communities, and educating children differently cannot be left to women alone.

Women will naturally remain the leaders and drivers of this work. I will always remain a voice for others. But women's rights are universal rights. When there is a petition, a demonstration, or a social media campaign about sexual violence, or an opportunity to talk about gender, sex, or inequality at home, men need to get involved. The problem concerns all of humanity, not half of it.

10

LEADERSHIP

Over the course of my career, I've met with many leaders of all different types: politicians, religious figures, business executives, community and grassroots organizers. There have been some who were closed to understanding the issue of sexual violence for reasons of personal ambition or misguided conviction, who choose to ignore or deny its existence. There have been many good ones, who are working to improve the lives of survivors and women generally, putting the values of compassion and kindness at the heart of their action. And there has been everything in between: people who are uncommitted, the wavering, the superficial or half-hearted.

Without all the leaders of any given society pushing in the same direction, it is very hard to produce the sort of systemic and cultural change needed to make the world a safer, more equitable, and more fulfilling place for women. Ending sexual violence can be achieved only through effort at every level. We need more leaders to be bold about using their influence.

In 2018, I traveled to Iraq to meet a leader whose community, like mine in eastern Congo, had been devastated by sexual violence. He had been forced to grapple with the consequences of a war on women's bodies, too. In a moment of huge adversity for him and his followers, he found the courage to challenge traditions and encourage profound social change.

My trip to Iraq was organized by a charity called Yazda, which has been working with the Yazidi community since 2014 and in particular with the women who suffered under the despicable and murderous rule of ISIS. The three-year hold of these extremists over northern and western Iraq left a trail of physical destruction that will take decades to repair.

When I flew to Erbil in northern Iraq, I had already met Nadia Murad, who had been working over the previous three years to raise awareness internationally about the targeting and mass rape of Yazidi women by ISIS, but my trip to Iraq occurred before we were both awarded the Nobel Peace Prize. Her bravery in sharing her story, first at the UN, then in media interviews, and then in her book, *The Last Girl,* means the infamy of this sickening chapter has been recorded for posterity.

ISIS was formed from the remnants of extremist groups such as al-Qaeda, which had battled American forces during the US occupation of Iraq from 2002. In early 2014, they overran the Iraqi army in northwest Iraq and gradually increased their sway until they controlled around a third of the country, including the country's second-largest city, Mosul, and the area around Sinjar, which is the historic heartland of the Yazidi community.

The Yazidis are a distinct ethnic and religious group whose origins can be traced back to the twelfth century when an Islamic mystic began preaching in the village of Lalish amid the mountains and scrubland of northern Iraq. Over centuries, his followers moved away from Islam, with the faith fusing with ancient local beliefs as well as drawing inspiration from Christianity and Judaism. It became a separate religion in its own right, with its own scripture, calendar, and ceremonies.

For more than eight hundred years, the Yazidis were caught in the battle for spiritual dominance that still grips the Middle East and large parts of the world today. They were a small minority that was preyed on and persecuted. Successive waves of oppression dispersed believers across the world.

Their survival as a community, numbering around five hundred thousand today, was due to the strong personal bonds between devotees, their religious piety, and the inhospitable terrain of their homeland, which includes the Sinjar Mountains, a mile-high ridge that over the centuries has offered refuge during each round of maltreatment.

Their targeting by ISIS was the latest attempt to wipe them out, only in the twenty-first century it was accompanied by a modern propaganda machine that the brutalized ancestors of today's Yazidis could never have imagined. Following the example of all genocidal ideologues, ISIS leaders dehumanized the Yazidis in their teachings and instructions, describing them as devil worshippers and apostates in their online messages and videos.

They began a campaign of mass extermination that drew in Nadia's family. Her village of Kocho was overrun in August 2014 at dawn by militants flying the sinister black flag of the group. After a week of cowering in their homes, everyone was called to the local school. The men, after being forced to hand over all their valuables, were separated from the women and children, lined up in front of a ditch, and shot in cold blood. Once the firing stopped, women and children, many sobbing hysterically, were loaded onto flatbed trucks together and driven to the ISIS-controlled city of Mosul.

Nadia, unmarried and then twenty-one, was selected to be a *sabiyya,* or slave wife, and driven at night on a bus to a market. "Every moment with ISIS was part of a slow, painful death," she wrote of the experience. The bus ride to the market, when she was molested and abused, was the "moment she started dying."

At the market—in reality a large room in a looted house—cruel, brutish, bearded men with guns arrived holding fistfuls of dollars. Many of them wanted to know if the girls were virgins. Nadia and her relatives screamed, rolled into balls, or tried to slap away the rough and callused hands that reached out to touch them. An estimated sixty-four hundred Yazidi women were traded like this into a sickening life of captivity.[1]

Nadia was sold to an ISIS judge who took sadistic pleasure in insulting her religion, forcing her to convert to Islam (which she pretended to do), and raping her repeatedly. He used to taunt her that even if she did escape, her life was over because her community would never accept her back. When she tried to flee and was caught, he ordered his guards to rape her as punishment.

She was sold on several occasions afterward, with none of her captors showing any sympathy as her health deteriorated. After three months, she managed to flee, taking advantage of an unlocked door, and she found shelter with a brave family of Sunni Muslims.

When I visited Iraq two and a half years later, ISIS had lost much of its territory in Iraq and in neighboring Syria thanks to the efforts of the Iraqi military, local militias including Yazidi and Kurdish fighters, and Western firepower provided by the United States and allies. But there was only the beginning of an effort to deal with the humanitarian crisis sparked by the fighting.

The first stop of my journey was at a refugee camp in Dohuk, a two-and-a-half-hour drive from the city of Erbil in an area controlled by the regional Kurdish government that had never come under ISIS control. Every few miles we needed to stop at checkpoints where we showed our papers and visas to groups of armed Kurdish guards.

In Dohuk, there were hundreds of thousands of displaced people housed in desperate conditions that were sadly familiar to me. Around 85 percent of the Yazidi community had been displaced by the fighting. The hills were dotted with camps, more arid and dry than ours in Congo but containing the same improvised architecture and markers of catastrophe found around the world.

Most people were housed in prefabricated homes rather than the tents found in refugee camps in Congo, and I was impressed by the solar panels and water tanks donated by the UN and aid agencies. Everything else I recognized: the daily scramble for food and water, children in worn-out clothes, parents with dead eyes watching over them.

There were thousands of women like Nadia there, victims of atrocities and rape who had had little or no professional care or support. A handful of doctors did their best to cope. The charity Yazda had asked me to visit to share our experience in Congo, hoping to learn from our approach in providing medical care as well as psychological, legal, and socioeconomic support. Sharing our expertise internationally has been a focus of my work in recent years.

They had arranged a meeting in one of the larger buildings with around fifty survivors who had volunteered to meet me. My hosts had told me before of their daily efforts to help the women in the camps who suffered from panic attacks, insomnia, and hysterical crying. Many had been rejected by their families. Others had borne children from their rapists. There had been suicide attempts.

The more I travel and learn, the more I realize that women suffer the same consequences of sexual violence, in the same way, in conflict zones and in peacetime, irrespective of their culture, language, or religious beliefs.

The group meeting made clear the scale of the needs for skilled psychological help and treatment. The trauma experienced by the women was still fresh and profound. Several women began recounting how they had been separated from their families by ISIS fighters, then were transported, sold, raped, and abused.

Once freed, they encountered a new set of problems. They were unable to return to their shattered homes and felt stigmatized by their community. Under Yazidi traditions, rape was viewed no differently than adultery. It was shameful for the victim. It could result in public floggings and murder at the hands of their relatives.

Nadia recounts how the first man who bought her used to tell her that as a raped Yazidi woman who had converted to Islam, her life was over. "Even if you make it home, your father or your uncle will kill you," he would sneer. She has described in candid terms her feelings of apprehension and fear when she did finally travel home.

As the women confided in me, it became obvious that their words were having an effect on others in the room. This is something we see frequently in Panzi during the first group therapy sessions. Women with untreated and suppressed traumatic memories can experience vivid flashbacks to their own ordeals. This is why "trigger warnings"—in which people are warned of upcoming references to sexual abuse—have become commonplace during public discussions about rape.

Four of the women fainted almost simultaneously. I attended to them, and once they were conscious we moved them to a quiet room where they could recover. I asked my hosts if there was a psychologist who could visit them afterward. There wasn't, I was told.

It demonstrated to me just how much work needs to be done to improve our emergency humanitarian responses during or after conflicts. The priority is naturally the urgent provision of food, shelter, and basic medical care. All too often, the invisible wounds of sexual violence go untreated, even though we know they exist.

Our next stop was the town of Lalish, to meet the leader I referred to in the introduction to this chapter. His name was Baba Sheik, the spiritual guide of the Yazidi people, a frail man of more than eighty with a long white beard.[2] He lived among the fluted, conical-shaped temples and natural springs in the community's religious capital.

All visitors have to remove their shoes before entering the village. It was a curious sensation to be walking barefoot over smooth cobblestones in streets shaded from the bright sunshine by thick mulberry trees.

I had been looking forward to meeting Baba Sheik, because in late 2014, as ISIS ransacked Yazidi villages, he decided to reinvent centuries of religious tradition. He concluded that compassion trumped theological dogma despite the risk of upsetting the traditionalists in the community.

After meeting several women who had passed through ISIS slave markets, he issued a decree to community elders that victims of the extremists should be welcomed back and should not face any consequences. Even more bravely, he declared that the babies delivered by these women as a result of their rape should be treated as Yazidis.

This contradicted one of the tenets of Yazidism. It is a closed religion. The community does not accept converts, and anyone who marries outside the faith is cut off. Women have been killed by relatives in the past for relationships with Muslims.

After Baba Sheik's announcements, Yazidi women raped by ISIS fighters began making pilgrimages to Lalish to be re-blessed with holy water found in one of the caves where all Yazidi children are baptized. They were given white head coverings as a symbol of rebirth. Many have returned several times, finding it a form of acceptance that helps them overcome their feelings of isolation and shame.

Baba Sheik sat cross-legged in his white robes when we met, and I touched my right forearm with my left palm as I bent over to shake hands, a sign of respect in Congolese culture. I explained why I was visiting Iraq and thanked him for receiving me. I shared how much I admired his decision and bravery in helping the women overcome the stigma of their experiences.

He was modest and self-effacing, insisting it was nothing radical and that the religion was simply evolving in the circumstances. Rejecting the women would merely be serving the interests of ISIS, whose objective was to destroy the community, he explained.

The decision was wise, humane, and progressive. All religious leaders, the guardians of the customs and beliefs that shape the lives of Christians, Muslims, Jews, and all our many faiths, have the capacity, and I believe the responsibility, to make our societies more accepting and welcoming places for women. They hold the spiritual and moral power to make a difference.

Change must come from the top in order to energize and influence those at the bottom. As I have stated repeatedly, sexual violence is a result of the gender hierarchy that holds male lives to be superior to female ones. We must acknowledge the role of religion in enforcing male dominance and female submissiveness.

I say this as a Christian and the son of a pastor. I am also a pastor at a small church in Bukavu in my father's parish. Some people around me have lost their ability to believe, concluding that it was impossible to reconcile the idea of a beneficent God who would watch impassively over two decades of slaughter in Congo. Without my faith, I know for sure that I would not have been able to continue all of these years.

I start each day with prayer focused on the values I find most important: love, compassion, humility toward God and all others, integrity, and solidarity. I go to church whenever I feel it is safe enough to attend. My Bible is my most cherished travel companion.

My relationship with God is a profoundly personal one. In fact, I consider myself to be a believer, but not necessarily a religious person. Religions are ideological constructions, interpretations of founding texts by significant figures of the past. These interpretations are the work of men, and they have usually used their positions of power to entrench their privileges.

We can decide whether to accept these interpretations as fixed, immutable laws laid down as firmly as the stones of the Lalish temples, the Wailing Wall, Mecca, or our cathedrals and churches. Or we can accept that dogma, too, must evolve, just as our celebrated religious buildings have been sometimes rebuilt, modified, expanded, shaped by the weather, and altered by human touch over time.

In my preaching in church, I have always insisted that the best place to meet God is inside ourselves, in our inner thoughts and consciences. Everything outside of this intimate sanctum is the work of humans, with all of their imperfections and vices. God for me is at the beginning and end of everything, a universal force that explains the inexplicable, including the perfection of nature, music, or art, and that urges us to love and care for one another.

Despite all I have witnessed of humans' capacity for selfishness and harm, I still believe that we are inherently virtuous, created in God's image, with vanishingly few exceptions. One must only stop to observe very young children in their innocence, their playfulness, and their purity to believe this. Their goodness, their saintliness, is true human nature before it is transformed by society, by rules and codes, and—let us be frank—sometimes by pernicious religious practices. Only inside of ourselves can we meditate on and renew our link to our original qualities, in dialogue with God.

I find no conclusive evidence in Christian scripture that women were born as inferior beings to men or that they should be subjugated. Adam was created and then Eve, who was formed in order that man should not live alone. They were created as a team, on the understanding that no animal would be their equal.

And I see no reason for other exclusionary and discriminatory practices against women, such as preventing them from taking positions of responsibility. The Gospel of St. Paul—most famously the line in First Corinthians that "women should remain silent in the churches"—has been used to justify a ban on women exercising power in the church. Given that there were several women leaders of the early church, colleagues of Paul, this phrase has almost certainly been misinterpreted and taken out of context.

I firmly believe that religious leaders must look to encourage, not resist, the wider societal changes underway that have seen the role of women across the world reevaluated over the last century to give them greater autonomy and power. History gives us countless examples of how religions have adapted to their times.

Feminism and faith are compatible concepts. The guardians of our temples, churches, and mosques should not feel threatened. That is why Baba Sheik's decision moved me so much. He had the clarity of mind and courage to recognize the need for change.

Sadly, in 2019, hard-liners within the Yazidi Supreme Spiritual Council issued a new statement clarifying that the children born from the rape of Yazidis would not be accepted, forcing survivors to make an impossible choice between their community and their offspring. The ordinance trickled down to community elders, who are tasked with enforcing the rules, complicating the lives of hundreds of women.

Traditional forms of leadership, sometimes elected figures but often assemblies composed of male elders, hold huge sway over the behavioral norms in vast areas of the world. They often take their cues from religious leaders, but it's important not to neglect the role they play in influencing attitudes and behavior, particularly in countries that are more collectively organized than highly individualized developed countries.

One of the major mistakes foreign aid organizations have made over the years in developing countries is neglecting or deliberately trying to bypass this essential level of society, which is often highly conservative. For example, I have witnessed aid groups and activists working on contraception trying to educate women directly about its benefits, without taking into account the social stigma attached to using it or the inability of women to make choices without the consent of their husband and the wider community.

Groups working on eradicating female genital cutting have for years focused their energies on changing laws and information campaigns, presuming that greater knowledge about the serious health risks associated with this practice and legal protections would be sufficient to bring it to an end. I have worked in Guinea in West Africa, where the vast majority of women continue to be subjected to cutting despite the law forbidding it.

Until community leaders—usually elders who act as spiritual and social arbiters—turn against it, the women found at the very bottom of the social hierarchy have negligible ability to make their own decisions. Indeed, many of them actively support cutting, seeing it as a coming-of-age ritual or even a bonding exercise between the women in a family.

The problems are the same when working on almost every women's welfare issue, from child marriage to polygamy.

Our work on promoting "positive masculinity" with the Warega tribe in South Kivu demonstrated to me that community-level change on women's rights can be achieved with gentle and respectful encouragement. It showed what can be achieved by working through existing power structures, not against them.

Following our initial training programs and seminars aimed at encouraging a more equal sharing of household responsibilities in their community, I was invited by the Warega elders to make a trip to their region in 2017. It was a sign of their gratitude and recognition of the relationship we had built up over several years. The aim of our visit was to discuss what else we could do for them and inspect some of the changes on the ground.

I was greeted there by the tribal chiefs, who are seen as providing the link between the Warega community and the spiritual world of their ancestors. In the absence of a functioning justice system, they are also expected to set the rules, adjudicate in disputes, and offer guidance to the community.

I spoke at the church first and went to visit a school that we had been funding. During our walk around the village, one of the elders confided in me about an embarrassing problem they had recently encountered with a foreign aid worker.

Over several years, the area had benefited from funding and help from a Western humanitarian organization that sent out staff to live and work among the tribe. In recent months, one of them, a German, had transgressed some of their strict rules designed to protect the dignity of their women, the elder explained.

The young man had been spotted in the bushes taking photographs of local women at a point on the nearby river that was a designated as a female bathing area. Men were strictly banned from this area, to allow the women to wash in privacy. Whether the young man was seeking a voyeuristic thrill or was capturing "exotic" images of local life to show relatives and friends back home was unclear.

The scandal reached the elders, who called a meeting. They were asked to decide how the community should react and whether the young German should be punished.

The elders ruled that he should be expelled from the village and must never return. He was exfiltrated in a hurry by his employers.

When we all sat down together at the end of my trip, I decided to use the story as a means of opening up a discussion about how to protect women in the community. We were all crammed into a space belonging to a local association working on sexual violence. The chiefs sat shoulder to shoulder on wooden benches, accompanied by their wives.

I began by stating something sincerely believed by everyone in the room: that the Warega prided themselves on protecting their women. Their decision to punish the German showed the extent to which they took their responsibilities to shield them from harm seriously. I recalled how their traditions also celebrated the role of mothers.

This is how many community leaders—whether in the Hindu caste *panchayat* in rural India, the *jirga* of Pashtun groups in Afghanistan or Pakistan, tribal assemblies in Africa, or Islamic clerics in the Middle East—see themselves. Treating them as ignorant misogynists closes down the space for collaboration and the sorts of discussions that can lead to change.

I told them there was something I needed them to explain to me: I understood that the German had committed a *muzombo,* a sin that was considered an outrage against the ancestors of the tribe. He had been sanctioned for a crime against local women by looking at them in the nude. But why were there not the same punishments for men who touched or penetrated women without permission?

I knew that the elders were often called upon to settle cases where men had been accused of raping girls and women in the area. Often, if the victim had been an unmarried virgin, the elders would offer the attacker a solution: pay her dowry and marry her. The issue would then be settled, with the "honor" of the girl's family—and supposedly her own—protected.

These so-called amicable arrangements are commonplace. Girls are simply traded: their fathers transfer ownership of their daughters to their rapists.

This has a perverse effect on local young men. If their marriage proposals are spurned by their desired spouse, they often resort to rape, knowing that in the rush to protect her "honor," they will be offered a face-saving opportunity to achieve by force what they were unable to accomplish with romance and charm. It's a powerful incentive for sexual violence that exists in many areas of Africa and around the world.

In other cases I had been told about, if the raped woman was married, the attacker would be ordered to make a payment to her husband, either financial or in livestock, with goats and chickens sometimes exchanged to settle a case.

"You have rules that forbid men from looking at women other than their wives in the nude," I said. "But shouldn't someone who has raped or molested another woman be treated more harshly than someone who has only seen?" I asked the elders. "You sanctioned this German man by expelling him, but shouldn't rape also be treated in the same way as a *muzombo*?" I continued.

Several of the elders explained that they took violence against women seriously and that they considered it a problem. The payments and "amicable arrangements" were, in their eyes, meant to deter aggressors.

"But you are punishing the girl. She is the victim of the crime and then you are forcing her to marry her attacker. You are doubling her pain," I argued. "Only if you declare rape a *muzombo* will it be a deterrent. No one will dare touch a woman without permission if they know they will be expelled."

Some of them objected, raising the problem of the girl's lost virginity and her honor. If she did not marry her attacker, she would find it very difficult to find another husband. This was true and a legitimate concern.

But I insisted that the elders could show leadership. "By speaking out against rape, you can help transfer the shame from the victim to the attacker. He is the one who should face difficulties, not her," I said. "And a more severe punishment would help prevent the crime in the first place. You would be saving others from this fate."

If I had flown in and begun lecturing the elders about their customs, I know I would have failed. But I knew they were acting in good faith. We had built up a relationship of trust, which meant they didn't take me for a university-educated doctor from the city who looked down on them. We had enough empathy for each other to create a space to exchange.

As we sat tightly packed in the room, the discussion about women and sexual violence went back and forth. I could tell that we were making progress. Some of them openly questioned their interpretations and could see the contradiction in how they punished voyeurism and sexual assault differently. By the end, all of them were prepared to see the need for rape to be declared a *muzombo* as well.

After we left, the elders reconvened and decided that they

would issue a decree that would be spread throughout the area—to the hundreds of thousands of people living in the dozens of villages under their sway. Rape was a crime that would now be punished with expulsion. There would be no more "amicable arrangements."

Like Baba Sheik in Iraq, they could see the need to question the traditions handed down by previous generations. They demonstrated what can be achieved by dialogue and a progressive mindset. They were prepared to question their assumptions and correct the errors of the past. My country, and the world more broadly, needs more leaders like the Warega elders.

On the other end of the spectrum, far removed from my travels to remote areas of eastern Congo, I have also, over the last decade and a half, interacted with world leaders and representatives of our global institutions. I have witnessed how we have collectively made progress in recognizing that sexual violence is a problem deserving of attention and action.

In 2008, two years after my first trip, I traveled to New York again at a time when the UN Security Council was discussing what would turn out to be a landmark resolution on the use of rape during conflicts. I was asked to brief the diplomats of the countries that make up the council, the five permanent members—the United States, China, Russia, the United Kingdom, and France—and ten others.

"Why are we talking about rape as an issue at the Security Council?" the Russian ambassador objected at one point during the discussions. He couldn't see how it was related to the body's mission of maintaining peace and preventing conflicts. I'm pleased to say I no longer encounter this sort of resistance. Rape is now accepted as being a consequence and often a deliberate tactic in all wars.

UN Resolution 1820, which passed unanimously in 2008 despite initial Russian skepticism, was an occasion that raised hopes of firmer action against the perpetrators of sexual crime in places such as Congo. It recognized the jurisprudence established by the international war crimes courts for Rwanda and Yugoslavia, which I referred to in chapter 7, acknowledging that rape could be used as a weapon of war and could constitute a war crime, a crime against humanity, and an act of genocide. It created obligations on states to investigate and prosecute perpetrators, and it also called for the deployment of more women in international peace missions.

The problem, like so many UN resolutions, is that well-intentioned words have not led to actions. There is no evidence that sexual violence in conflict zones has diminished as a result of the months of intense diplomatic negotiations that led to the vote in favor of Resolution 1820. Armed forces or militias committing rapes in Congo, Sudan, Myanmar, or Syria still enjoy the same impunity.

A year later, the UN Security Council passed another important follow-up resolution, 1888, which created the Office of the Special Representative of the Secretary-General on Sexual Violence in Conflict, a welcome development that has helped focus attention on the issue.

In the decade since then, the UN Security Council has steadily passed further resolutions—seven in all—on women and security, including Resolution 1960, which established a monitoring and reporting mechanism on sexual violence in conflict, and Resolution 2106, which again stressed the need for accountability.

The work has been vital in spreading awareness, but Russia and China remain skeptical about the expansion of the women and security agenda at the UN, while the Western alliance, which has been the driving force behind the progress, was put under unprecedented pressure by the actions of the Trump administration.

In 2019, when the German government put forward another resolution, number 2467, about rape in conflict zones, the Trump administration threatened to veto it if it included any reference to the importance of rape victims having access to sexual and reproductive health services—on the grounds that this implied access to abortions.

This backsliding on previous resolutions, which had stated the importance of access to health services such as HIV checks as well as emergency contraception if requested by a survivor, was a reminder that nothing can be taken for granted. Momentum built up over the last decade looked as if it were going to be lost.

In the end, a compromise was found in a watered-down version that removed any reference to sexual and reproductive health services, as well as to the vulnerability of gay, lesbian, and transgender people in conflicts. I took satisfaction from the fact that the resolution made reference for the first time to the importance of a survivor-centered approach to caring for the victims of sexual assault and also recognized the need to support children born of rape. The US voted in favor. China and Russia abstained.

In late 2020, Russia tried again to weaken the gains made over the last twenty years with a new resolution that would have diluted some of the previous commitments. Fortunately, its resolution, backed by China, was easily defeated by the other members.

There have been other national-led efforts to combat sexual violence. Former US president Barack Obama, the British government under Prime Minister David Cameron, Prime Minister Justin Trudeau of Canada, and latterly French president Emmanuel Macron have all made contributions. Sweden became the first country in the world to pursue a "feminist" foreign policy in 2014 under a male prime minister, Stefan Löfven, based on three Rs: rights, representation, and resources.

In 2014, the British government also organized the first ever Global Summit to End Sexual Violence in Conflict. Hosted by then British foreign secretary William Hague and actor and activist Angelina Jolie, it brought together policy makers, survivors, civil society groups, and experts. I attended, as did three members of the Congolese government, which I saw as an encouraging sign.

Hague and Jolie visited Congo in the run-up to the conference, visiting the village of Minova, which was the scene of mindless violence by government troops in late 2013. Having just lost a battle with the Rwanda-backed M23 rebels, they went on a two-day drunken rampage of raping and looting. One soldier later told journalists that he and twenty-five comrades got together and decided they would rape ten women each.[3]

The problem with summits is the same as the problem with UN resolutions. They help focus attention for a brief time on the issue, but they often fail to follow through on their ambitions. I remember a meeting with Prime Minister Cameron in which he questioned how the British government was going to sustain its efforts after the summit, which cost £5.2 million (nearly $7 million) to organize.

I went home from the event feeling that it lacked substantive conclusions. There was little progress on the issues I sought to highlight in my speech, such as the need for sanctions on governments that protected or failed to prosecute perpetrators of sexual violence. The UN resolutions needed to be given teeth, I argued. Unless there were consequences, leaders would continue to ignore them.

A highly critical independent review by the government's aid watchdog published in 2020 found that the conference had "not fully delivered on its ambitions and is at risk of letting survivors down." It highlighted the lack of political leadership after Hague's departure as foreign secretary, as well as dramatic cuts in funding for the agenda in the six years since the meeting.[4]

Leadership to promote the women's rights agenda internationally is essential and necessary, but the scope for change is limited unless UN resolutions are enforced or the International Criminal Court is expanded and empowered. Our supranational legal mechanisms remain weak. Only national leaders have the ability to change discriminatory laws, invest in the police and judicial resources necessary to prosecute perpetrators, and promote real social change through their speeches and personal example.

In order to make governments more responsive, we need more women in positions of power. We need more female leaders capable of breaking through the glass ceilings that prevent them from reaching the presidencies, prime ministerial offices, and chancelleries from which they have been historically excluded.

I was struck while attending the G-7 meeting of the world's richest nations in France that when the leaders posed for a group photo, the only female political officeholder was Angela Merkel of Germany. During her decade and a half in power, she often found herself as the sole woman at the table during meetings of the twenty-eight-member European Union or at the Group of 20 (G-20) international summits.

When granted the keys to power, women are more likely to make the changes we need to make our world fairer and safer. When they are given a platform, they can use the opportunity to prioritize issues important to them, such as maternal rights, more equal pension systems, education, or more accommodating workplaces that take into account the different needs of women compared with men. And these changes do not serve women alone; they help children, husbands, and fathers, too.

In my experience, I've always found that when women succeed, they do not succeed for themselves. They share that success easily with their husband, their children, and their community. This makes them more willing to weigh up the collective, rather than the personal, when making decisions. Men tend to be more driven by their own concerns of personal wealth, success, and ambition.

Women often bring skills lacking in their male counterparts. It was striking how many of the countries that won the most praise initially for their handling of the novel coronavirus crisis from their fellow citizens were run by women, such as Germany, New Zealand, Denmark, Iceland, and Norway.

It would be overly simplistic to suggest, based on this evidence alone, that gender was an important factor in determining how governments reacted. It is tempting to think that managing the crisis played to the traditional strengths of women managers, who are often better at teamwork and displaying empathy than their male peers. Conversely, the macho populist strongmen, who refused to heed advice from experts and admit the limitations of their own knowledge, were among the worst performers. In any case, the crisis was an important victory for an argument that sadly still needs to be made in the twenty-first century: that women make equally competent political leaders as men, if not better, and can be trusted with power.

The latest statistics from UN Women show just how unequal political leadership remains at the global level. There are only around twenty women heads of state or government around the world out of 193 nations surveyed, according to the latest data.[5] A 2019 study by the OECD found that only four out of thirty-six leading democracies had achieved gender parity in their governments—Canada, France, Sweden, and Slovenia. The average in all thirty-six nations was one women for every three men in ministerial posts.[6]

The *Global Gender Gap Report* produced by the World Economic Forum measures four things to assess the differences between men and women in the 153 countries it studies. These include equalities in economic opportunities, education, health, and politics. The biggest gap globally is in political empowerment.

In its 2020 report, it found that only 25 percent of 35,127 parliamentary berths globally were occupied by women. It noted improvements in the last twelve months. But even if progress were sustained at this level, it would still take 94.5 years to close the gender gap in political representation.

The more women are in politics, the more they are able to address historic gender imbalances. And the more they open up pathways for other women to follow them, the more they will succeed in making politics a safer, more respectful place. Because chauvinism and sexual abuse are rife in our parliaments and councils, too.

In 2016, the first international study of sexual harassment and violence against female lawmakers, by the Inter-Parliamentary Union, found that 82 percent of women parliamentarians polled had experienced some form of psychological violence. Twenty percent had been sexually harassed. A follow-up study in 2018 focused on members of parliament in Europe confirmed the same levels of abuse in the European Union and also revealed that 40 percent of female parliamentary staff who took part had been sexually harassed at work.

We should all be concerned about a relatively new trend of women abandoning their political ambitions because of the difficulties they have, in dealing not just with the macho internal culture but with the level of misogynistic abuse directed at them over social media by men. Ethnic-minority women are particularly in need of support.

The senior ranks of the business world are just as imbalanced as our parliaments. The OECD compiles statistics for the number of women who sit on the boards of the largest publicly listed companies. They found that in the thirty-six leading democracies worldwide, women on average held only one in four seats. The share of female managers was only slightly higher, at around one in three.

The proportion of female board members has increased sharply from a very low base in the last fifteen years, in some countries owing to legislative pressure. Norway became the first country in the world to oblige companies to name at least 40 percent of women on public and state-owned company boards. France, Italy, Spain, and the state of California have since followed suit with mandatory quotas. An alliance of major investors called the 30% Club is pushing for that proportion of women on boards.

Many studies have highlighted the benefits of gender-diverse boards, showing that women can help check the overconfidence of male CEOs, stopping them from overpaying with acquisitions,[7] or improve corporate governance and the quality of discussions about strategic decisions.[8]

Wherever women are promoted, they help to break down the historic masculine norms of most organizations. In my personal experience, men tend to behave better when there are women around. They curb their tendencies to be arrogant, combative, and overbearing.

A major study from the McKinsey & Company consultancy in 2018 called *Delivering Through Diversity,* which analyzed one thousand companies in twelve countries, concluded that businesses with a higher proportion of women in leadership positions, as well as a mixed ethnic and cultural composition, delivered higher profitability and longer-term value for shareholders.

There is another area where women's involvement is crucial,

which is close to my heart as a citizen of a war-ravaged country: they are still dramatically underrepresented in peace processes, and yet their participation has been shown to positively affect the likelihood of the guns falling silent for good.

In peace negotiations from 1992 to 2019, only 13 percent of negotiators, 6 percent of mediators, and 6 percent of signatories to peace agreements were women, according to a study by the Council on Foreign Relations, a US think tank.[9]

A separate study in 2015 found that when women participate in peace processes, the resulting agreement is 35 percent more likely to last at least fifteen years.[10] Female peace negotiators were also found to be more likely to include provisions for women, such as a recognition and compensation for sexual abuse.[11]

This was certainly the case for Colombia, which in 2016 succeeded in producing one of the most gender-sensitive peace agreements ever signed. Women's civil society groups and women representatives were included in the process with FARC rebels from the start by President Juan Manuel Santos. They helped secure compensation mechanisms for victims, a commitment that sexual crimes would not be amnestied, and a pledge that judges tasked with trying war crimes in a special court would be made up equally of men and women.

They have also pushed for the creation of a center for survivors offering medical, psychological, and socioeconomic help modeled on the "holistic" approach we take at Panzi Hospital, and have succeeded in securing public recognition for the more than fifteen thousand women who suffered sexual assault during a conflict that lasted fifty years.

A new art installation in Bogotá called *Fragmentos* features a floor formed from thirty-seven tons of rifles turned in by rebels as part of the peace agreement. The weapons were melted down by artist Doris Salcedo, who invited rape survivors to help pound the metal into tiles with mallets. The effect is stunning—I found it immensely empowering to be walking on destroyed weapons, as Salcedo intended—while the production process was also apparently cathartic: women felt they were hammering away at their traumas while working.

I admire the creativity, thoughtfulness, and commitment to include women in the Colombian peace process. If only we could rely on the same enlightened thinking in Congo. To conclude this chapter, I want to tell you more about the difficulties I have faced with my own government.

I have described previously the naked threats and intimidation I have suffered. I want to describe the only time President Kabila came to my hospital, which helps explain why so little has been done to recognize, care for, and protect the women of Congo over the last twenty years.

Kabila visited in 2010, his ninth year in power. His appearance was prompted not by outrage over the constant influx of injured women and girls at this time but by an accident involving a petrol tanker in the village of Sange around forty-five miles south of Bukavu. It had overturned and a crowd of people had rushed forward to collect fuel in plastic bottles. It exploded, killing 269 and injuring more than 200. Many of the most complicated cases and severe burn victims were transferred to Panzi Hospital.

Kabila announced a national day of mourning, and his staff contacted me to say he planned to visit the region and see some of the survivors. I notified the staff that we would finally be receiving a long-awaited presidential visit.

He pulled up in the parking area in a shiny black 4x4. I stood waiting to greet him, with the hospital staff behind me. His door was opened for him and he stepped out. We shook hands.

"Welcome, Your Excellency, and thank you for coming," I said. I searched his face for signs of emotion. I found only hardness as he scanned the scene in front of him silently.

"Thank you. . . . You know why I am here, don't you?" he said as we moved toward the hospital.

"Yes, Your Excellency, of course."

"Why have I come, then?" he continued, speaking to me as a headmaster might address a pupil.

"You've come to visit the burn victims. My staff have been working flat-out," I said.

"Yes, that's right. I'm not here to see your women."

Your women. I needed to concentrate hard to keep my composure. The callousness of his words, the way he had dismissed the survivors in the hospital, the patronizing way he had questioned me: he seemed to ooze contempt. I knew many women were waiting at that moment back in the survivors' center. They wanted an opportunity to speak with him, to draw attention to the toll of the conflict on their lives and communities.

I took him to the ward where some of the burn victims lay in their beds, heavily bandaged. He greeted several of them, offering his condolences. There was a rattle of clicking noises. The gaggle of press photographers captured the moment of him leaning in sympathetically over their beds.

"Did you receive the supplies I asked to be sent from Kinshasa for the injured?" he asked, returning his attention to me when we paused in the middle of the room. There were more clicking noises. Boxes with burn dressings and treatments had been sent for all the hospitals caring for the wounded in the region, he informed me.

"We received a box," I explained. "But I'm afraid it was of no use."

"Why?" he replied sharply.

I paused momentarily. I knew the answer would be embarrassing for him. "It contained acetaminophen, condoms, and medicine for intestinal worms," I said.

"How is this possible?" he snapped. He turned around and glared at his entourage, who looked grave and uncomprehending. One of them jotted down a note.

It needed no explanation. We all knew what had happened. It's the story of modern Congo, the gangrene that explains why our army and police are without vehicles, uniforms, and ammunition for their weapons. It's why roads and public buildings are half-built and teachers go unpaid. It's why our airlines have appalling safety records and our banks go bankrupt, gobbling up people's life savings in the process.

He had probably released some money to buy medication and ordered that it be sent to the hospitals. But the first person who received the order would have taken a cut of the money, then the second and the third, perhaps all the way down to the final person packing the box. At some point, the small quantity of medical supplies actually purchased had been stolen and sold on the black market. But something had to be sent. Appearances had to be kept up. So condoms and acetaminophen were packed instead.

When he'd finished touring the ward for burn victims, I ignored his opening remarks at the car and suggested that he visit the sexual violence wing anyway. His mood seemed to darken further. He reminded me curtly again why he was there.

As we continued our walk back toward his car, I felt more and more frustrated. As he made to get into his vehicle, I made one final appeal.

"Your Excellency, it is such a shame for you to come all this way and not visit these women who have suffered so much," I said, fixing his eyes with mine. "Please take the time, even if it is only to greet them quickly."

His eyes narrowed under his brow and his face stiffened. "It's of no interest to me. This problem will be sorted in six months. This hospital won't be here anymore," he shot back, gesturing with a slight flick of his head toward the buildings behind us.

What to make of these sinister words? I expected him to get inside his car at once and slam the door. I was again lost for words. But to my surprise, he paused and looked behind us.

"What's that over there?" he asked, glancing toward a separate building where we care for malnourished children. "I'll look in there," he said.

I agreed to give him a quick tour. There were rows of beds with children in them, anxious mothers at their side, in a facility we had set up shortly after opening the hospital. It is always full, despite Congo having some of the most fertile earth in Africa.

At the end, in a final flourish of what had been a profoundly discouraging and unsettling experience, he promised me some money for the children. The next day, the regional governor arrived with journalists and photographers in tow to hand me $50,000 in cash wrapped in a brown paper bag. He didn't ask me to sign anything and left no instructions about how it should be spent.

Kabila earned himself some positive media coverage. His visit was reported in the local and national media, with pictures of him in the ward. His cash donation for the hospital was duly published, too.

But why the resistance to visiting the women? Was it self-preservation? Did he believe that acknowledging the mass rape of women in Congo was something personally dangerous, given the responsibility of the state and the fact that sexual crimes can be prosecuted under international law as a war crime?

Possibly. But it is more likely that he simply resorted to the instinctive desire to cover up something he viewed as shameful and embarrassing. He preferred not to engage with it. He'd rather the women stayed silent and me, too, even if that meant closing the hospital, the only specialized medical center for sexual violence in the region. It was a total abdication of leadership.

As the years went by after his visit, I became more, not less, outspoken. The hospital has never closed. There was never any attempt to do so in the six months after.

Again and again throughout Kabila's misrule, I could never understand why the international community did not do more to pressure him into carrying out the necessary work of reforming the Congolese security forces, tackling corruption, and improving state services, which might have brought an end to the instability.

The smuggling of the minerals that sustains the fighting has continued, along with the money laundering by Congolese politicians and their cronies through overseas shell companies and properties acquired in European cities. Foreign interference and the funding of militias on Congolese soil remains a problem.

I witnessed what can be achieved with sufficient political will in

2012. For the first time, Rwanda faced serious international pressure over its support for the ethnic Tutsi M23 rebel group, which was responsible for mass rapes, executions, recruiting child soldiers, and displacing hundreds of thousands of people in eastern Congo.

When the UN concluded in a report that the rebels were being controlled by the Rwandan government, President Obama called on President Kagame to cut off the logistic and political support. The United States, the United Kingdom, Germany, the Netherlands, Sweden, and the European Union all froze or threatened to cut off their military and budgetary aid to Rwanda. The effect was almost instant: M23 was liquidated. Its head, Bosco Ntaganda, ended up at the International Criminal Court and is now behind bars.

As for Kabila, only at the end of his time in office, as he rode roughshod over the constitution in an attempt to cling to power from 2016, did the European Union and the United States impose asset freezes and travel bans for the first time on people around him. A bolder, more assertive approach earlier on would have produced results.

The errors of the past cannot be repealed, but they can be repaired.

At the end of 2018, Congo voted in delayed and fraud-tainted elections for a new president. Opposition figure Félix Tshisekedi, son of veteran pro-democracy campaigner Étienne Tshisekedi, emerged as our new leader. But in disputed parliamentary elections held at the same time, Kabila's party managed to win a majority and retain its grip on power amid widespread claims of cheating. It has created an uneasy and potentially destabilizing power-sharing arrangement.

Foreign leaders must support efforts for justice and accountability in Congo. The anarchy and more than five million dead and missing constitute one of the most overlooked, underreported, and neglected conflicts of the modern era. Much of the violence and economic plundering has been documented already.

Each passing year of violence in eastern Congo, each ransacked village, each new admission of a shattered body in my hospital, adds to the ongoing tragedy of my country. It is sick. It needs to heal. Doctors like me have picked up the pieces, repaired bones, and stitched up bloodied wounds for too long.

And what is true for Congo is true for the cause of women's rights: if you are in a position of power and influence, you can help. And if you're not working for a solution, you're part of the problem.

CONCLUSION

We all face moments when we doubt ourselves, when we question our choices and feel like giving up. The costs can sometimes seem too high, the effort not worth it. I have experienced many such occasions over the years, often after periods of particularly harrowing work or during long sleepless nights. I found myself at a crossroads in late 2012.

It followed events at my house on a cool evening in October when two women came knocking, just as the sun was setting at around six P.M. At that time, we lived in a bungalow located not far from Lake Kivu, separated from the dusty, unpaved road outside by a high concrete wall topped with razor wire. We'd moved there because it was the safest area of Bukavu. The headquarters of the UN peacekeeper force was just down the road.

I had grown accustomed to receiving patients at home. Lots of them knew where we lived, and sometimes, when they couldn't make it to the hospital five miles away, they'd come to the gate of the compound and ask for me. The guards knew to let them in if I was at home.

It was a mother and daughter. The older one had a swollen and infected foot. When I'd finished examining her, she asked if I could drive her to an area of the city where they could find one of the creaking Toyota taxi vans, all rust and battered bodywork, that serve as our public transport system.

I was shattered, having just returned from a trip to Europe. I was on edge and my insomnia had returned. I'd received some threatening phone calls and messages again, something that seemed to happen every time I went abroad to try to raise awareness about the conflict.

But the woman's infected foot made walking visibly uncomfortable for her. I agreed to drive them and backed our car out of the driveway. I left my two youngest daughters, then fifteen and seventeen, and their cousin, inside.

After a journey of no more than twenty to thirty minutes, there and back, I returned home. I gave two short beeps of the horn in front of the house, the usual signal that I was outside. Then came the first indication that something was perhaps wrong.

A young man I'd never seen before opened the door of the compound and stuck his head out to look at my car. It was unusual, but not necessarily a cause for alarm: the guards would occasionally invite friends over, and they'd sit in their cabin, chatting or playing cards to pass the time. Maybe a friend had been sent to check it was me.

The metal gate slid open, scraping on its wheels and shaking as it pulled back to reveal the empty courtyard behind. Night had fallen by now. The beam of the headlights struck the wall of the house in front of me. Then there was sudden movement.

I saw the silhouettes of five men with long shadows dart toward me. Before I had time to react, they were around my vehicle. The doors were flung open. One jumped in the front, four in the back. The one beside me pressed the tip of a machine gun against my stomach. One of the men in the back—I couldn't turn to see his face—held a pistol to my temple.

My first thought, which surged forth at the same time as a burst of adrenaline, was of a university professor in Bukavu who'd been killed just months before like this, by men who had broken into his house. It was another unsolved crime, like most of the murders.

Was I going to die like him? Maybe. Or was it a carjacking or a robbery, which would mean I had a chance of surviving? Or was it people carrying out one of the death threats against me? One thought raced into another, each one sparking a fresh inquiry. Could I escape? Probably not. If I couldn't escape and was going to be murdered, could I kill some of them before they started firing?

The concrete wall of the house was a distance of around thirty feet from the car. I made a split-second decision. If I accelerated hard and rammed us into it, without seat belts, I figured my at-tackers would be thrown violently toward the windshield. It might seriously injure them.

I pressed the accelerator. But as the car lurched forward, I was struck by a second contradictory impulse: What about the pastor friend of mine who'd been abducted in Goma at the other end of Lake Kivu a few weeks back? He'd been driven around for three hours, his hands bound behind his back, before being dumped by a cemetery, traumatized but uninjured. It was a warning, not an attempt to take his life.

I hit the brakes. The car heaved; everyone lurched forward with the momentum. The wall of the house was no more than three feet away when we came to a stop. "You're not going to kill us, are you?" said the man with the machine gun in Swahili. It was the only time I heard him speak.

He reached across and snatched the keys out of the ignition. The man with the pistol in the backseat ordered me out of the car. The front door of the house was now a short stretch away. If I could get out and run, maybe I could save myself. Safety seemed within reach.

I opened the door, swung my legs around, and was about to make my move. But the man with the Kalashnikov in the front seat had walked around the car and moved in front of me, barring the way, his finger on the trigger. They weren't interested in my car, then, I thought. This was an assassination. I saw him ready his weapon.

There was something about the icy look in his eyes. And the men seemed too disciplined, too organized, to be a gang of thieves. As I stood there helplessly, I thought of Madeleine, how she'd left earlier in the evening to attend a friend's wedding without me. I felt a nauseating bolt of panic as I imagined my daughters inside.

I thought of the number of times I'd escaped death in the past, the occasions when I'd fled just in time or had been called out of harm's way. My luck had run out here; my intuition about danger had deserted me. How many people had died in Congo like this, facing the indifferent stare of a cruel young man with a gun?

Just at the moment that I was bracing for the bullets, I heard a shout.

A man tore around from the side of the building, screaming and waving his arms. It was one of our employees at home, Joseph. He'd been tied up by the gunmen but had managed to wriggle free and had been watching from the shadows. As he burst forward in a desperate bid to protect me, he must have known he faced almost certain death.

I can still hear him shouting—"Papa! They're going to kill you!"—and the rattle of the bullets that struck him at close range as he approached me. I don't remember what happened next. I passed out. He slumped over in a heap, between the car and the front door. Our bodies must have fallen almost simultaneously. His blood pooled on the driveway and seeped into my clothes.

After opening fire, the gunmen fled in my car. They probably assumed the shots had alerted the police and the UN forces nearby. They needn't have worried—neither arrived until the following day.

The next thing I remember was stumbling, dazed, into the house. My daughters had been held at gunpoint inside. One of the men had kept watch over them, saying nothing other than "If you want to live, keep quiet." They'd offered him money and jewelry to leave, but he'd refused with a shake of his head.

They had kept quiet, waiting for my return with their backs against the wall facing the driveway, terrified about what was in store for me. If I had crashed the car into the house, as I'd first thought to do, I'd probably have killed them.

"Papa, get down!" they screamed as I lurched into the house, trembling and in shock.

I've played over the events of that evening a thousand times and it is still not clear how I survived. Did the gunmen think I had been hit when I collapsed next to Joseph? Did they mistake his blood for mine? I will never know.

I will also never know who sent them. Someone in neighboring Rwanda? A warlord in eastern Congo? A high-up in the army or someone else from the Congolese state? Was it linked to my recent public appearance at the UN?

The year before, at the Waldorf Astoria in New York, I'd been threatened by the then health minister, who had warned me I would be in danger if I went ahead with a planned speech at the UN. As I described in chapter 6, I'd backed off and canceled, feeling as if I had been silenced like so many victims of sexual violence.

In 2012, just a month before the attack at my home, I'd taken a calculated risk: I was again invited to address a UN panel on sexual violence during the General Assembly. This time I accepted and spoke.

There was no real attempt to find my attackers. A few police officers arrived on the scene afterward. They looked around lazily, snapped a few photos, but none took witness statements, not even a description of the men, who had made no attempt to hide their faces. No prosecutor visited. Joseph was buried without anyone examining his body. My car was found abandoned a few days later.

At police headquarters in Bukavu, I saw in news reports months afterward that investigators had a cardboard file with "Dr Muk-wege case" scrawled on it in pink marker. A senior officer showed it off to journalists, including the handwritten notes inside detailing their "hypotheses." No one has ever been arrested.

Two days after the attack, I drove with Madeleine and my daughters to the airport in silence. I was once again fleeing Bukavu, heading to an unknown life overseas. This was the final straw. I felt sure that if we stayed, we were in grave danger. I felt completely exposed.

Local UN forces had agreed to escort us to the airport. Their armored vehicles—one in front, three behind—made it feel like an evacuation. This was the end, I felt. For thirteen years since 1999, I'd worked on the rape crisis in eastern Congo and had never lost my determination to keep the hospital running, to continue operating day after day, and to speak out.

The gunmen changed my calculations. My responsibility as a parent and a husband weighed heavily on me, eclipsing the sense of duty I had for the community and the patients I served. And what good would I be to anyone riddled with bullets, lying in a grave? Like Joseph. Dear old Joseph.

We flew to Brussels and then on to Sweden, to the company of friends and colleagues. I wondered throughout what our life would be like. Would I be able to work remotely and keep up my campaigning?

During our first week in Europe, an organization I'd worked with in the past, Physicians for Human Rights, came to our rescue. They offered to fly me, Madeleine, and my youngest daughters, Denise and Lina, to Boston and they would provide us with a house. I remain immensely grateful for their help.

Our lodgings in the United States offered a new level of comfort. The kitchen was huge and modern. A beautiful wooden staircase climbed from the living room to an upstairs hallway, with doors opening out into five bedrooms, all en suite. The house needed no security guards, no razor wire.

We arrived in the middle of a bitterly cold winter, with snow on the ground. I sketched out a six-month plan in my mind: if we were going to make a success of our American life, we needed to learn English as a priority. We enrolled the children in school, and Madeleine and I began taking intensive language classes from morning until the late afternoon.

After about three weeks, the spare room came in handy. Our dear friend Jean Lebel, a pastor from Bukavu who had been a constant source of support and encouragement over the years, came to visit. Seeing him gave me an instant connection to what we had left behind. His kindly face was familiar and warm. And he brought news that filled me with pride and joy.

A group of women on the island of Idjwi in Lake Kivu, a few hours' journey by boat from Bukavu, had written to President Kabila. In their letter, they demanded that the government bring me back and provide security for me so that I could continue my work. Jean brought me a copy of the letter in his bag, with hundreds of signatures affixed to a typeset page.

I barely knew the island of Idjwi, although I'd treated many women from there. I grinned, then broke into stunned laughter. President Kabila had no interest in my work with the women of Congo, as he had told me so memorably during his visit to the hospital. This letter couldn't possibly make a difference.

But two weeks later, after Jean had headed home, I got a call from the hospital in Bukavu. The women had written again, this time to the UN secretary-general. A few weeks after that, the women came to the hospital in person.

"They turned up today and told us that you absolutely had to come back," my colleague Magambo informed me over the phone.

"That's incredible, but do you think they're serious?" I asked.

"They said they would pay for air tickets for you and the family if you'd agree to come back. They even promised to guard the hospital. They said twenty-five of them would stand outside at all times and no one could get to you."

"That's . . . ridiculous," I said. "You don't believe it, do you?"

Most of these women lived on less than a dollar a day and could barely pay for their own families, let alone four air tickets from the northeastern coast of America to central Africa.

"They said they'd come here every Friday until you come back," Magambo continued. "And they're going to sell food in front of the hospital to raise the money."

And the following Friday they were true to their word. After taking the ferry with baskets of fruit and vegetables, they appeared outside the hospital, setting up stalls along the road and selling pineapples and passion fruit, eggs, corn, and cassava.

I've often wondered why it was the women of Idjwi. There was no particular reason, no bond with them stronger than that with any of the other communities we served across the region. But every social movement has to start somewhere, and they took matters into their own hands.

It was too much for me. In the following weeks, women joined in the campaign from across South Kivu. Some traveled through rebel territory, from Bunyakiri where Mai-Mai fighters still terrorize villages as well as from Kahuzi-Biéga National Park or Kavumu.

The balance started to tip. I began to weigh up the thousands of women back home and my work there against the duty of protection I felt toward my own family. One evening a few days after Christmas, with the snow piling up in the garden, I shared what I was contemplating at the dinner table.

"I think I should go back to Congo, but you should stay here in Boston," I announced. They all looked up from their food in silence. "It's not safe for you there, but I can come back here for long periods and during the holidays. We can work something out," I added.

The idea filled my daughters with dread and a desire to protect me. The youngest, Denise, from the height of her fifteen years, was the most adamant.

"It was you they were looking for, not us, when they came to the house," she said. "If anyone should stay here in Boston, it's you. No way are you going back on your own. If you go, we all go."

She was so categorical, so determined, I found it hard to argue. I'd spent my life admiring the strength of the women of my region. Now my own daughter was growing up before my eyes, possessed of the same determination.

We talked some more. I continued to make the case for only me to return, but it was no use. From then on, there was an inevitability about our return.

At one moment or another, all activists living and working in a dangerous part of the world face a moment like this, when they must ask themselves whether they are prepared to die for their cause. After the attack in October at my home, I hadn't been—fear had gotten the better of me. But as I thought about the spontaneous market by the women of Idjwi, I realized I was prepared to give up everything for them. Death would be senseless. But so would a life lived in the comfort of Boston.

In mid-January, three months after leaving, we went back.

The final leg of the journey saw us take a flight home from Bujumbura in Burundi. I was seated at the window as the single-propeller Cessna climbed and banked northward, following the route of the Ruzizi River toward Bukavu. Madeleine was at my side, our daughters behind.

Our whole lives had played out in this part of Africa, in places strung along the tormented land below us. I'd done my first medical studies in Bujumbura. Madeleine and I had lived there as a newly married couple and started our family there.

We flew over the hills surrounding Lemera Hospital where I'd first discovered the suffering of mothers without access to health care, over the forests I'd gone hiking in and the road I'd taken just days before the outbreak of the First Congo War for a terrifying journey that saved my life. The hospital and the mass grave dug for my murdered patients were down below around halfway through the flight.

The toll of conflict since the attack on Lemera Hospital in 1996 was clearly visible on the ground. To the east of the river lay Burundi and Rwanda. I could see farmers there working their strips of land. On the Congolese side on the west bank, where there had once been fruit plantations, fields of cotton, and rice fields, the land was now untended.

I was lost in these melancholy thoughts about the waste and the potential of Congo as Bukavu loomed into view below. The atmosphere in the plane had been tense since we'd taken off; everyone seemed to be preparing themselves. I could sense Madeleine's nerves. We were exchanging the freedom of the United States for a life in Congo that risked being even more uncertain and claustrophobic than ever.

We held hands. I needed her as I've needed her at every step in our more than forty years of marriage. We're like two trees that hold each other up by leaning together, our branches intermingled.

"It'll be okay," I said. It was a half-hearted attempt at reassurance. We both knew what we were going back to. The only thing I could really count on was her love and support. That had been enough to get me through the toughest moments of the past.

The plane descended. As we bounced down the airstrip, I got my first glimpse of what awaited. Stepping down from the plane, I saw a ring of UN peacekeepers keeping hundreds of well-wishers back. I managed to greet my mother and a few members of my family before the crowd rushed forward.

The road from the airport, which had seemed so desolate when we had taken it in the opposite direction months before, was now lined with people waving and celebrating our return. When we arrived back at the hospital, it was packed. Staff had organized a welcome-home ceremony. We had to push our way to a stage that had been put up in one of the courtyards.

It was draped with blue-and-white fabric, with chairs arranged in three neat rows. Behind the microphone at the front, there was a seat for me and one for the governor of the province, Marcellin Cishambo, whom I had known since childhood. As I sat looking out at the crowd in front of us—hospital staff, patients, men, women, and children—it was hard to forget how he had gone missing when I had needed him after the attack in October.

To my right, on the end of the second row of seats onstage, was the regional police chief, his dark navy uniform immaculate, his jaw set firm. His display of support was hardly reassuring. As long as I didn't know who wanted me dead, it would be impossible to feel safe.

The ceremony felt formal and insincere—right up to the moment that the mothers and grandmothers of Idjwi gate-crashed the party.

They arrived with shrieks and ululations. Heads turned, the signboards and banners in the crowd twitched; part of the crowd shifted, then parted. A group of a few dozen of them, some carrying children on their backs, pushed past the chairs and up to the stage. They wanted the microphone, which was passed down.

I didn't recognize any of them. One by one, they spoke. One by one, they denounced the government and the police for failing to prevent crime and their inability to stop gangs and militias preying on communities in the province.

"If you won't protect the doctor, then we will!" said one woman who was pushed up to the stage in a wheelchair, gesturing toward the governor and the police chief. "Tonight there will be twenty-five of us guarding the hospital, and if someone wants to kill the doctor, they will have to kill twenty-five defenseless mothers first!"

In between their speeches, they sang and they clapped. "Dr. Mukwege, Doctor, stand up! Dr. Mukwege, have you seen him standing up?" they sang. "Don't try to touch him, or we'll knock you to the ground!"

All the while, women were coming to the front of the stage to empty their baskets and pots. There were onions for me, pineapples and pumpkins, too. One woman had brought a turkey. Each of them handed over a welcome-home present.

My throat grew tight, making it hard to swallow and impossible to talk. Tears filled my eyes. I knew in every fiber of my body that I was back where I belonged—among them.

I composed myself and stood up to speak to bring an end to the ceremony. Someone brought me my white doctor's jacket, which I swapped for my suit. Just as I finished, the weather broke and giant raindrops began rattling the roofs of the hospital buildings and splashing down on the leaves of the surrounding trees. Everyone ran for shelter.

That moment with the women of Idjwi was a turning point in my life. It was a moment of profound communion with my patients. I had spent my professional life working for the women of eastern Congo, and at exactly the moment I felt at my lowest ebb and at my most vulnerable, they had flown to my side.

I felt that I understood their experiences more than ever, even though I had tasted only a fraction of what they had endured. I had felt the helplessness and fear of being overpowered by someone else. I had been deprived of my freedom, forced to submit, and humiliated. And I knew the burn of injustice after experiencing a violent crime that no one was interested in investigating or solving.

This is the fate of every woman who suffers sexual violence. The difference is that I escaped with my body intact. My ordeal lasted only minutes. I was not molested or penetrated. I do not have physical scars to remind me of that awful evening at my home.

The women of Idjwi treated me instinctively as we should treat all victims of crime, but especially victims of sexual violence. They sent me a message, in the form of their letter, to reassure me that I was not alone, that they had my back, that they understood my pain. It felt like an embrace or a reassuring arm across my shoulders.

As individuals and as societies, we need to show this sort of compassion and kindness to all survivors. Sadly, instead, we tend to do the opposite. We compound their pain by treating them with suspicion, or worse, treating them as pariahs. The shame and costs of an assault all too often fall on women, not their aggressors. They deserve sympathy, support, and protection.

I am sure you, the reader of this book, knows someone in your family, or in your personal or professional circles, who has needed an arm across a shoulder at some point. Or perhaps you have read or heard about someone whose story has touched you. Always reach out. A small amount of your time could make all the difference. Empathy has the potential to transform our world.

The women of Idjwi also demonstrated the power of the collective. As an individual, I had been frightened and intimidated. Yet they drew strength from each other. They felt emboldened because they linked arms.

Only collectively can we smash the taboos around sexual violence, ensuring that it is something that is openly discussed and tackled, not swept under the carpet like a dirty secret. This is why the campaigns of recent years—from SlutWalk to #BringBackOur-Girls to #MeToo—need to be applauded and encouraged.

But awareness campaigns aren't enough on their own. They are great at generating publicity. They can thrust an issue or person into the spotlight. But they can't help a woman who needs assistance in filing a police complaint. They can't lodge a case against a negligent or insensitive investigator. They can't offer counseling or a safe place to stay for the victim of an abusive partner or family member.

These tasks are often handled by grassroots women's organizations that need support. The women of Idjwi formed a collective that did more than just write letters. They mobilized. They turned their emotions into action. You can play a role, too, by supporting or offering your time to local groups helping victims of domestic or sexual violence.

Finally, in order for real change to occur around the world, we need people like those who sat next to me on the stage during the ceremony at the hospital—the police chief and the governor, people with responsibility and power—to hear and take on board the messages addressed to them. We need more female police chiefs and governors, too.

Women are speaking out in ever greater numbers around the world to demand respect and security, just as the women of Idjwi did when they demanded the microphone. Mindsets must change. Sexual violence should be a public policy priority. Our criminal justice systems have to improve. Rape needs to be criminalized in reality, not just on paper.

You can play a role in a variety of ways to help make the world safer for women. Support others. Speak out. Join or help a collective. Build pressure on your elected representatives and law enforcement. And play a role as an educator by using your knowledge.

We are all educators to the people around us: to children, friends, and family, to colleagues or team members. Call out sexism. Condemn and report predatory behavior. Push back on victim blaming. Explain the impact of stigma and trauma. Ensure that opportunities in your family or workplace are equally distributed between men and women, girls and boys.

And don't forget to teach the boys around you to be respectful, so that we don't have to protect our daughters. If your role is as a community educator—as a journalist, historian, teacher, or professor— your potential to serve as a force for positive change is greater than most. And if you are a politician or a faith or community leader, remember that your words and actions—as well as your silences and inaction—have the capacity to harm or heal.

I have never regretted returning home in 2013. I decided to continue working in a place where I feel the most useful and fulfilled. We are all at our most useful and fulfilled when we look beyond ourselves and ask what we can do for the less fortunate, the oppressed, the ignored.

Women and victims of sexual violence in particular have been oppressed and ignored for most of human history. Every one of us can be useful in correcting this injustice, driven not by a desire for revenge on men but by a desire for empowerment and security for all.

After the ceremony at the hospital, I went to live in a new home. Madeleine and I didn't feel safe enough to return to our bungalow in the center of Bukavu where I had been attacked. Instead, we moved into one of the original buildings of the Panzi Hospital compound, one of the old colonial-era cottages that we had renovated fifteen years earlier to turn into an operating theater. We converted it back into a house.

I live there now, under permanent armed guard. I have a dozen UN peacekeepers stationed outside twenty-four hours a day. They serve as my armed escort every time I leave the hospital, though I rarely venture out. I thank them every morning for their presence as I make the two-hundred-yard trip from my front door to the rest of the hospital.

I am quite sure that without their protection I would be dead. Only my trips abroad relieve the feeling of being a prisoner in my own home, and the Nobel Peace Prize in 2018 was not the game changer you might imagine. It has given me a higher public profile, but the lawlessness in eastern Congo, the diffuse and varied threats against me, and the recent political changes leave me with a constant sense of vulnerability.

But there will be no letup in my campaigning to amplify the voices of women around the world. I try to channel at all times the directness and impact of the young girl who brought an army general to his knees before me. I am driven on by the bitterness I feel when remembering Wakubenga, who was attacked twice and infected with HIV, or the woman whose daughter and granddaughter were both born through rape. I am constantly inspired and uplifted by the resilience of my former patients Bernadette, Jeanne, Alphonsine, and Tatiana, among many others.

I will also continue to spread the expertise and knowledge we have built up in Bukavu in treating victims of rape in conflict zones. In numerous areas of the world, survivors find themselves abandoned, as I witnessed while visiting the camp of Yazidi families in northern Iraq a few years ago. We can help deliver specialized medical care, psychological assistance, and social and economic support.

In Congo, the Panzi Hospital and Foundation, thanks to the work of its staff and support from our generous donors, continues to expand and find new ways of helping survivors. Our microfinance initiatives are growing. We have a new clinic and shelter in the capital, Kinshasa. We have even started a fresh juice business in Bukavu, processing the passion fruit, pineapples, and oranges grown on our farm, run by survivors.

My greatest hope is that one day our wards and shelters for raped women will fall empty, that our counseling services and lawyers' offices will become obsolete. I hope that I and my staff might dedicate much more of our efforts to the work that first inspired me as a student doctor in the 1980s: the marvel of childbirth and maternal health.

My happiest moments are still at our maternity center, seeing the rows of exhausted but smiling mothers and hearing the faint cries of infants. When we look down on a newly born child, everything seems to stop still for an instant, forcing us to reflect on what sort of world we want them to grow up in.

I pray every day for a peaceful and prosperous future for my country and region. We are rich beyond belief in nature and resources, yet greed and exploitation have made us one of the poorest places on the planet. Still today, villages are burned to the ground and massacres take place every week with barely a ripple of indignation in and outside Congo. We need justice and accountability.

I dream of a society in which our mothers are recognized as the heroines they are, in which the girls born on our maternity wing are celebrated just as much as the boys, and in which women grow up without fearing violence.

I hope for a world where women have the same opportunities for professional advancement and personal joy and fulfillment as men and where political power is shared equally. I can't wait for the day when our businesses and public institutions reflect the diversity of the societies we live in. I also imagine a future when sexual assault is seen as a throwback to an earlier, more brutal era.

I believe all of this is both desirable and possible. I believe that we can all make contributions as individuals and as collectives to make it happen. I believe in the power of women.

ACKNOWLEDGMENTS

$\mathcal{I}$t will come as no surprise to you that, when contemplating whom to thank for this book, my thoughts immediately turn to the patients and incredible women I have described in these pages. They deserve the highest praise and my most sincere gratitude.

But deciding whom to feature, whose story to tell, was a difficult process. I was able to introduce only a fraction of the hundreds of survivors who have left their mark on me during conversations in my consulting room or on the wards of the hospital. I want to thank each of them for their trust.

I must also acknowledge the incredible hard work and commitment of the staff of the Panzi Hospital and the Panzi Foundation. Their devotion to serving our community saves lives, heals wounds, and lifts people back to their feet every single day. And they do this while facing the daily hardships of life in Bukavu. Christine Amisi, who heads the foundation, and Christine Schuler Deschryver from the City of Joy deserve special praise for their unrelenting energy.

Tineke Ceelen was the first woman I discussed the idea of this book with—and I will always be grateful to her for her unswerving commitment to victims of sexual violence.

I would like to thank my literary agent, Susanna Lea, who helped make this book happen. She believed in it from our first meeting and has championed it tirelessly at every turn since.

Thank you to Oprah Winfrey, Bob Miller, and Bryn Clark, my editor at Flatiron Books, for their enthusiasm and help in bringing this book to an American audience.

Thank you to Adam Plowright. Without his understanding, patience, and skill, I would not have been able to write this book.

And lastly, thank you to my wife, Madeleine, and my children, for being the lights of my life.

NOTES

1. MATERNAL COURAGE

1. Van Reybrouck, David. *Congo: The Epic History of a People*. New York: HarperCollins, 2014, 47.

2. A WOMEN'S HEALTH CRISIS

1. United Nations International Children's Emergency Fund. *State of the World's Children 2014 in Numbers: Every Child Counts*. New York: UNICEF, 2014. https://data.unicef.org/resources/state-worlds -children-2014-numbers-every-child-counts/.
2. UN Inter-agency Group for Child Mortality Estimation. "Stillbirth and Child Mortality Estimates." New York: IGME, 2021. https:// childmortality.org/.
3. Delivery care data from UNICEF. https://data.unicef.org/topic /maternal-health/delivery-care/.
4. GBD 2015 Maternal Mortality Collaborators. "Global, Regional, and National Levels of Maternal Mortality, 1990–2015: A Systematic Analysis for the Global Burden of Disease Study 2015." *Lancet* 388, no. 10053 (October 2016): 1775–1812. https://www.thelancet.com /journals/lancet/article/PIIS0140–6736(16)31470–2/fulltext.
5. Ibid.
6. Centers for Disease Control and Prevention. "Pregnancy Mortality Surveillance System." https://www.cdc.gov/reproductivehealth /maternal-mortality/pregnancy-mortality-surveillance-system.htm.
7. Pregnancy-Associated Mortality Review Project Team. *Pregnancy-Associated Mortality, New York City, 2006–2010*. New York: New York City Department of Health and Mental Hygiene, Bureau of Maternal, Infant and Reproductive Health, n.d. https://www1.nyc.gov/assets /doh/downloads/pdf/ms/pregnancy-associated-mortality-report.pdf.
8. Organisation for Economic Co-operation and Development. *SIGI 2019*

Global Report: Transforming Challenges into Opportunities. Social Institutions and Gender Index. Paris: OECD Publishing, 2019. https://www.oecd-ilibrary.org/development/sigi-2019-global-report_bc56d212-en. Also see: International Labor Organization. *Maternity and Paternity at Work: Law and Practice Across the World.* Geneva: ILO, 2014. https://www.ilo.org/wcmsp5/groups/public/—dgreports/—dcomm/—publ/documents/publication/wcms_242615.pdf.

9. US Department of Labor. *National Compensation Survey: Employee Benefits in the United States, March 2019.* Washington, DC: US Bureau of Labor Statistics, 2019. https://www.bls.gov/ncs/ebs/benefits/2019/employee-benefits-in-the-united-states-march-2019.pdf.

10. Chzhen, Yekaterina, Anna Gromada, and Gwyther Rees. *Are the World's Richest Countries Family Friendly? Policy in the OECD and EU.* Florence: UNICEF Office of Research, 2019. https://www.unicef-irc.org/family-friendly.

11. Organisation for Economic Co-operation and Development. "Parental Leave: Where Are the Fathers?" Paris: OECD Publishing, March 2016. https://www.oecd.org/policy-briefs/parental-leave-where-are-the-fathers.pdf.

12. Stearns, Jason. *Dancing in the Glory of Monsters: The Collapse of the Congo and the Great War of Africa.* New York: PublicAffairs, 2011, 116.

13. Rapaport, Lisa. "U.S. Relies Heavily on Foreign-Born Healthcare Workers." Reuters, December 4, 2018. https://www.reuters.com/article/us-health-professions-us-noncitizens/u-s-relies-heavily-on-foreign-born-healthcare-workers-idUSKBN1O32FR. Patel, Yash M., Dan P. Ly, Tanner Hicks, and Anupam B. Jenna. "Proportion of Non–US-Born and Noncitizen Health Care Professionals in the United States in 2016." *Journal of the American Medical Association* 320, no. 21 (2018): 2265–67. https://jamanetwork.com/journals/jama/article-abstract/2717463.

3. CRISIS AND RESILIENCE

1. The Community of Pentecostal Churches in Central Africa was founded by Swedish Protestants.

2. Peterman, Amber, Tia Palermo, and Caryn Bredenkamp. "Estimates and Determinants of Sexual Violence Against Women in the Democratic Republic of Congo." *American Journal of Public Health* 101, no. 6 (June 2011): 1060–67. https://ajph.aphapublications.org/doi/10.2105/AJPH.2010.300070.

4. PAIN AND POWER

1. "The Congo Literacy Project (the Democratic Republic of Congo)." Hamburg: UNESCO Institute for Lifelong Learning, February 2020. https://uil.unesco.org/case-study/effective-practices-database-litbase-0/congo-literacy-project-democratic-republic-congo#:~:text=Programme%20Overview,women%20in%20the%20Mennonite%20community.

2. *Democratic Republic of the Congo, 1993–2003, UN Mapping Report.* Geneva: UN Office of the High Commissioner for Human Rights, Au-

gust 2010, 99. https://www.ohchr.org/Documents/Countries/CD/DRC
_MAPPING_REPORT_FINAL_EN.pdf.

3. Figures from Panzi Hospital patient records show 4.5 percent of patients were found to be HIV positive at this time.

5. IN HIS WORDS

1. Learning on Gender & Conflict in Africa (LOGiCA). *Sexual and Gender-Based Violence in the Kivu Provinces of the Democratic Republic of Congo: Insights from Former Combatants*. Washington, DC: World Bank, September 2013. http://documents1.worldbank.org/curated/en/795261468258873034/pdf/860550WP0Box380LOGiCA0SGBV0DRC0Kivu.pdf.

2. Figure based on accounts from diplomats and reproduced by Watchlist on Children and Armed Conflicts, a nongovernmental organization.

3. A full account of life inside an Alliance of Democratic Forces for the Liberation of Congo rebel boot camp near Lemera can be found in Stearns, *Dancing in the Glory of Monsters,* 145–50.

4. Ibid., 152.

5. Beevor, Antony. *Berlin: The Downfall 1945*. New York: Viking, 2002.

6. Judgment of the International Military Tribunal for the Far East.

7. *Report of the Panel of Experts on the Illegal Exploitation of Natural Resources and Other Forms of Wealth of DR Congo.* New York: United Nations Security Council, April 2001, 6. https://www.securitycouncilreport.org/atf/cf/%7B65BFCF9B-6D27–4E9C-8CD3-CF6E4FF96FF9%7D/DRC%20S%202002%201146.pdf. https://reliefweb.int/report/democratic-republic-congo/report-panel-experts-illegal-exploitation-natural-resources-and.

8. Zounmenou, David, Nelson Alusala, Jane Lewis, Virginie Monchy, and Bart Vanthomme. *Final Report of the Group of Experts on the Democratic Republic of the Congo*. New York: United Nations Security Council, June 2019, 36. https://www.securitycouncilreport.org/atf/cf/%7B65BFCF9B-6D27-4E9C-8CD3-CF6E4FF96FF9%7D/S_2019_469.pdf.

9. He refers to total population losses, including children who were not born because of the terror, of ten million. Three separate estimates arrived at roughly the same figure, including a Belgian government commission in 1919, a top executive of the Congo state, and a study by anthropologist Jan Vansina from the University of Wisconsin. Detailed in Adam Hochschild, *King Leopold's Ghost: A Study of Greed, Terror, and Heroism in Colonial Africa* (London: Macmillan, 1999), 253.

10. Thornton, William, and Lydia Voigt. "Disaster Rape: Vulnerability of Women to Sexual Assaults During Hurricane Katrina." *Journal of Public Management and Social Policy* 13, no. 2 (2007): 23–49. https://28b3dd4c-a-e2cc6547-s-sites.googlegroups.com/a/jpmsp.com/new-jpmsp/Vol13Iss2-DisasterRape-ThorntonandVoigt.pdf?attachauth=ANoY7coDrRktC6w8pB-AheSEeb5i-pirc48Wx3SjLFCRKiV5l7issbszi7NLIovPvLdq_hkdv9cBsLbmPXhEWjvhze2D1UFuQws8MhFVuJsOrz_SuZA_MgOUMFxY1BIMWCwQtPOdla_rOClnsJCLsAxOZRXsZGgn4

e0Fs0qCOXrR7ykXPcPCU4_jZfHIm8jmx_wzFGMQMBQW5BJbW5W
WrJztVImvUMXERZ0Xzwx_F-tB1Uuf0FhfpBA%3D&attredirects=0.

11. Smith, Sharon G., Xinjian Zhang, Kathleen C. Basile, Melissa T. Merrick, Jing Wang, Marcie-jo Kresnow, and Jieru Chen. *National Intimate Partner and Sexual Violence Survey: 2015 Data Brief.* Atlanta: Centers for Disease Control and Prevention. https://www.cdc.gov /violenceprevention/datasources/nisvs/2015NISVSdatabrief.html.

12. Crime Survey for England and Wales, 2017. https://www.ons.gov.uk /peoplepopulationandcommunity/crimeandjustice/bulletins/crimeine nglandandwales/yearendingmar2017#:~:text=Excluding%20fraud% 20and%20computer%20misuse%20offences%2C%20there%20 were%20an%20estimated,the%20year%20ending%20March%20 2017.

13. "Personal Safety, Australia: Statistics for Family, Domestic, Sexual Violence, Physical Assault, Partner Emotional Abuse, Child Abuse, Sexual Harassment, Stalking and Safety." Canberra: ABS, 2017. https://www.abs.gov.au/statistics/people/crime-and-justice/personal -safety-australia/latest-release.

14. Debauche, Alice, Amandine Lebugle, Elizabeth Brown, Tania Lejbowicz, Magali Mazuy, Amélie Charruault, Justine Dupuis, Sylvie Cromer, and Christelle Hamel. *Violence and Gender Relations (Virage) Study.* Paris: National Institute of Demographic Studies, 2015. https:// www.ined.fr/en/publications/editions/document-travail/enquete -virage-premiers-resultats-violences-sexuelles/.

15. World Health Organization Department of Reproductive Health and Research, London School of Hygiene and Tropical Medicine, and South African Medical Research Council. *Global and Regional Estimates of Violence Against Women: Prevalence and Health Effects of Intimate Partner Violence and Non-Partner Sexual Violence.* Geneva: World Health Organization, 2013. https://www.who.int/publications /i/item/9789241564625.

16. The *Report on Sexual Assault in the Military* has been running since 2006. https://www.sapr.mil/reports. https://www.sapr.mil/sites /default/files/public/docs/reports/MSA/DOD_Annual_Report_on _Sexual_Harassment_and_Violence_at_MSAs_APY19–20.pdf.

17. Pérez-Peña, Richard. "1 in 4 Women Experience Sex Assault on Campus." *New York Times,* September 21, 2015. https://www.nytimes .com/2015/09/22/us/a-third-of-college-women-experience-unwanted -sexual-contact-study-finds.html.

6. SPEAKING OUT

1. Bartels, Susan, Jennifer Scott, Denis Mukwege, Robert Lipton, Michael VanRooyen, and Jennifer Leaning. "Patterns of Sexual Violence in Eastern Democratic Republic of Congo: Reports from Survivors Presenting to Panzi Hospital." *Conflict and Health* 4, no. 1 (May 2010): 9–18. https://conflictandhealth.biomedcentral.com/articles/10.1186 /1752–1505–4–9.

2. Harris, Elizabeth A. "Despite #MeToo Glare, Efforts to Ban Secret

Settlements Stop Short." *New York Times,* June 14, 2019. https://www
.nytimes.com/2019/06/14/arts/metoo-movement-nda.html#:~:text
=the%20main%20story-,Despite%20%23MeToo%20Glare%2C%20
Efforts%20to%20Ban%20Secret%20Settlements%20Stop%20
Short,only%20one%20effectively%20neutralizes%20them.&tex-
t=Such%20agreements%20have%20been%20a,court%20settle-
ment%20for%20sexual%20misconduct.

3. Roughly 3 in every 100,000 women in Africa were killed by an intimate partner or family member, while 1.6 in every 100,000 Americans suffered the same fate, as did 0.9 per 100,000 in Asia. The Asian
figures in particular include wide discrepancies, with women facing
significantly higher danger in places such as Afghanistan, Pakistan,
and India. United Nations Office on Drugs and Crime. *Global Study on
Homicide 2019.* Vienna: UNODC, 2019. https://www.unodc.org/unodc
/en/data-and-analysis/global-study-on-homicide.html.

7. FIGHTING FOR JUSTICE

1. https://www.asil.org/insights/volume/14/issue/38/un-mapping
-report-documenting-serious-crimes-democratic-republic-congo.
2. Rape, Abuse & Incest National Network. "The Criminal Justice System: Statistics." Washington, DC: RAINN, 2021. https://www.rainn
.org/statistics/criminal-justice-system.
3. https://fra.europa.eu/sites/default/files/fra-2014-vaw-survey-at-a
-glance-oct14_en.pdf.
4. Research and Statistics Division. "JustFacts." Ottawa: Department of
Justice, Government of Canada, April 2019. https://www.justice.gc.ca
/eng/rp-pr/jr/jf-pf/2019/apr01.html.
5. Levy, Ro'ee, and Martin Mattsson. "The Effects of Social Movements:
Evidence from #MeToo." SSRN, March 2020. https://conference.nber
.org/conf_papers/f138191.pdf.
6. Barr, Caelainn, Alexandra Topping, and Owen Bowcott. "Rape Prosecutions in England and Wales at Lowest Level in a Decade." *Guardian,*
September 12, 2019. https://www.theguardian.com/law/2019/sep/12
/prosecutions-in-england-and-wales-at-lowest-level-in-a-decade.
7. Franceinfo. "Les condamnations pour viol ont chuté de 40% en dix ans."
France Télévisions, September 14, 2018. https://www.francetvinfo
.fr/societe/harcelement-sexuel/les-condamnations-pour-viol-ont-chute
-de-40-en-dix-ans_2940491.html.
8. Kelly, Liz, Jo Lovitt, and Linda Regan. "Gap or a Chasm? Attrition in Reported Rape Cases." London: Great Britain Home Office Research Development and Statistics Directorate, February 2005. https://webarchive
.nationalarchives.gov.uk/20110218141141/http://rds.homeoffice
.gov.uk/rds/pdfs05/hors293.pdf.
9. Kennedy, Pagan. "The Rape Kit's Secret History." *New York Times,*
June 17, 2020. https://www.nytimes.com/interactive/2020/06/17
/opinion/rape-kit-history.html.
10. Brand-Williams, Oralandar, and Kim Kozlowski. "10 Years In, Detroit
Rape Kit Crisis Vanquished." *Detroit News,* December 15, 2019. https://

www.detroitnews.com/story/news/local/wayne-county/2019/08/13/detroit-touts-success-rape-kits-crisis/3770362002/.

11. Rape, Abuse & Incest National Network. "Understanding Statutes of Limitations for Sex Crimes." Washington, DC: RAINN, n.d. https://www.rainn.org/articles/statutes-limitations-sex-crimes.

8. RECOGNITION AND REMEMBRANCE

1. Ungar-Sargon, Batya. "Can We Talk About Rape in the Holocaust Yet?" *Forward* magazine, April 25, 2018. https://forward.com/opinion/399538/can-we-talk-about-rape-in-the-holocaust-yet/.

2. Ibid.

3. Tanaka, Yuki. "War, Rape and Patriarchy: The Japanese Experience." *Asia-Pacific Journal* 18, no. 1 (December 2019): 1–14. See also extract in Tanaka, *Hidden Horrors: Japanese War Crimes in World War II* (Oxford: Routledge, 2018), 105–10.

9. MEN AND MASCULINITY

1. *Population Prospects: The 2017 Revision, Key Findings and Advance Tables*. Working Paper No. ESA/P/WP/248. New York: United Nations, Department of Economic and Social Affairs, Population Division, 2017. https://population.un.org/wpp/Publications/Files/WPP2017_KeyFindings.pdf.

2. Organisation for Economic Co-operation and Development. "Gender Wage Gap." Paris: OECD, 2021. https://data.oecd.org/earnwage/gender-wage-gap.htm.

3. *Global Gender Gap Report 2020*. Geneva: World Economic Forum, 2019. https://www.weforum.org/reports/gender-gap-2020-report-100-years-pay-equality.

4. El Feki, S., B. Heilman, and G. Barker, eds. *Understanding Masculinities: Results from the International Men and Gender Equality Survey (IMAGES)—Middle East and North Africa*. Cairo and Washington, DC: UN Women and Promundo, 2017. https://www.unwomen.org/-/media/headquarters/attachments/sections/library/publications/2017/images-mena-multi-country-report-en.pdf?la=en&vs=3602.

5. All figures are taken from the OECD's "Violence Against Women" database. https://data.oecd.org/inequality/violence-against-women.htm.

6. The United States has no federal legislation banning corporal punishment, which is allowed in public and private schools in nineteen states. Federal legislation has been repeatedly introduced in recent years without success, according to the campaign group End Corporal Punishment. For more information, see https://endcorporalpunishment.org/reports-on-every-state-and-territory/usa/.

7. Capraro, Valerio, and Hélène Barcelo. "The Effect of Messaging and Gender on Intentions to Wear a Face Covering to Slow Down COVID-19 Transmission." PsyArXiv, May 11, 2020. https://doi.org/10.31234/osf.io/tg7vz.

8. Sim, Shin Wei, Kirm Seng Peter Moey, and Ngiap Chuan Tan. "The Use of Facemasks to Prevent Respiratory Infection: A Literature Review in the Context of the Health Belief Model." *Singapore Medical Journal* 55, no. 3 (March 2014): 160–67. https://www.ncbi.nlm.nih.gov/pmc/articles/PMC4293989/.

9. Planned Parenthood. "PPFA Consent Survey Results Summary." New York: Planned Parenthood, 2016. https://www.plannedparenthood.org/files/1414/6117/4323/Consent_Survey.pdf.

10. Shammas, Brittany. "Judge Awards $13 Million to Women Who Say They Were Tricked into Pornography." *Washington Post,* January 3, 2020. https://www.washingtonpost.com/business/2020/01/03/judge-awards-million-women-who-say-they-were-tricked-into-pornography/.

11. Wright, Paul J., Robert S. Tokunaga, and Ashley Kraus. "A Meta-Analysis of Pornography Consumption and Actual Acts of Sexual Aggression in General Population Studies." *Journal of Communication* 66, no. 1 (February 2016): 183–205. https://academic.oup.com/joc/article-abstract/66/1/183/4082427?redirectedFrom=fulltext.

12. Rostad, Whitney L., Daniel Gittins-Stone, Charlie Huntington, Christie J. Rizzo, Deborah Pearlman, and Lindsay Orchowski. "The Association Between Exposure to Violent Pornography and Teen Dating Violence in Grade 10 High School Students." *Archives of Sexual Behavior* 48, no. 7 (July 2019): 2137–47.

10. LEADERSHIP

1. This figure was provided in 2018 from the Ministry of Religious Affairs of the regional government of Kurdistan in northern Iraq. Around half were known to have escaped or had been rescued, while the fate of the rest was unknown.

2. Baba Sheik, whose real name was Khurto Hajji Ismail, died in October 2020 at the age of eighty-seven. His honorific title has been passed to his successor.

3. Jones, Pete. "Congo: We Did Whatever We Wanted, Says Soldier Who Raped 53 Women." *Guardian,* April 11, 2013.

4. Review by the Independent Commission for Aid Impact, published January 2020. https://icai.independent.gov.uk/psvi/.

5. "Women in Politics: 2020." UN Women and Inter-Parliamentary Union, January 2020. https://www.unwomen.org/-/media/headquarters/attachments/sections/library/publications/2020/women-in-politics-map-2020-en.pdf?la=en&vs=827.

6. Organisation for Economic Co-operation and Development. *SIGI 2019 Global Report: Transforming Challenges into Opportunities.* Social Institutions and Gender Index. Paris: OECD Publishing, 2019. https://www.oecd-ilibrary.org/development/sigi-2019-global-report_bc56d212-en.

7. Chen, Jie, Woon Sau Leung, Wei Song, and Marc Goergen. "When Women Are on Boards, Male CEOs Are Less Overconfident." *Harvard*

Business Review, September 12, 2019. https://hbr.org/2019/09/research-when-women-are-on-boards-male-ceos-are-less-overconfident.

8. Gul, Ferdinand, Bin Srinidhib, and Anthony Ng. "Does Board Gender Diversity Improve the Informativeness of Stock Prices?" *Journal of Accounting and Economics* 51, no. 3 (April 2011): 314–38. https://www.sciencedirect.com/science/article/abs/pii/S0165410111000176?via%3Dihub.

9. Bigio, Jamille, Rachel Vogelstein, Alexandra Bro, and Anne Connell. "Women's Participation in Peace Processes." New York: Council on Foreign Relations, n.d. https://www.cfr.org/womens-participation-in-peace-processes/.

10. O'Reilly, Marie, Andrea O Suilleabhain, and Thania Paffenholf. "Reimagining Peacemaking: Women's Roles in Peace Processes." New York: International Peace Institute, June 2015. https://www.ipinst.org/wp-content/uploads/2015/06/IPI-E-pub-Reimagining-Peacemaking.pdf.

11. True, Jacqui, and Yolanda Riveros-Morales. "Towards Inclusive Peace: Analysing Gender-Sensitive Peace Agreements 2000–2016." *International Political Science Review* 40, no. 1 (2019): 23–40. https://journals.sagepub.com/doi/pdf/10.1177/0192512118808608.

INDEX

Access Hollywood, 232

Addis Ababa Fistula Hospital, Ethiopia, 79

advocacy, women's rights. *See also* legislation, rape; positive masculinity; prosecution of rape
  awareness campaigns as, 83, 127, 139–41, 143, 274
  via City of Joy institute, 92–5, 127, 160
  community support as tool for, 273–5
  corporate equity and, 175, 255
  diversity of representation in, 140
  by elders, 244–9, 275–6
  intimidation efforts against, 141–2, 143–7, 151–5, 165, 257, 264, 267
  via investigation/prosecution of rape, 156–86
  via legislation, xvi–xvii, 178–84, 217, 219
  via Maison Dorcas institute, 97, 149, 160
  media as tool for, 161, 186
  via MUSOs, 97, 99, 277
  NDA's interference with, 142–3
  parenting as tool for, xvii, 212–6, 227–35, 275–6
  peace process and, 256–7
  political parity and, 252–5, 278
  via positive masculinity, xvii, 31–2, 212–35, 245–9
  by religious leaders, 236, 241–4, 275–6
  survivor storytelling as, 90–1, 127–34, 138–9, 154, 173, 191–2, 198–200, 203–5
  by UN/global institutions, 249–52, 261
  by women, xii–xiii, xvi–xvii, 87–100, 252–7, 269–75

Affleck, Ben, 160

Afghanistan, 168, 186

African Americans, 33–4

African Union, 148

AIDS/HIV, xii, 89–90, 250, 277

Akayesu, Jean-Paul, 166

Alliance of Democratic Forces for the Liberation of Congo, 50

Allied Forces, rape by, 109, 202–3

Alphonsine (rape survivor), 93, 98–9, 277

American Families Plan, 34

Amisi, Christine, 97, 279

Annan, Kofi, 136
appetitive aggression, 104–7, 109, 121
Aristotle, 159
Association of American Universities, 124
Australia, 177, 200, 223
  rape statistics in, 123
  WW II rapes by, 202–3
Axios, 175

Baba Sheik, 236, 241–2, 244, 249
Bachelet, Michelle, 155
Badilika program, 222–6, 245–9
Ban Ki-moon, 154, 172
Batumike, Frederic, 159–63, 165, 186
BaziBaziba people, 13–8
Belgium, 182–3
  colonialism of, xiii, 2–17, 40, 54–5, 118–9
Bergman, Majken, 6–8
"Bernadette" (rape survivor), 67–70, 72–3, 205, 277
Biden, Joe, 34, 139
Black Lives Matter, 119, 218
Boko Haram, 210
Bolsonaro, Jair, 229
Bosnia and Herzegovina, rapes in, 109–10, 115, 166, 197, 203–5
Braeckman, Collette, 161
Brazil, 209
Breaking the Silence, 139
#BringBackOurGirls, 210, 274
British Commonwealth Occupation Force, 202
Brownmiller, Susan, 108
Bujumbura, Burundi, 25, 36–7
Bukavu, Congo, 11–3, 41, 43.
    See also Panzi Hospital, Bukavu, Congo
  geographical characteristics of, 8–10
  infrastructure of, 84–5, 220
  Mukwege's birth/childhood in, 1–8, 18–22
  war's impact on, 48–53, 54–7

Burke, Tarana, 140
Burundi, 14, 23, 43, 47, 49
  Congo Wars and, 50, 57, 106, 147, 170, 271
  medical school in, 25, 36–7, 271
Bush, Billy, 232
BVES charity, 120, 125–6

Cadière, Guy-Bernard, 79, 156
Cambodia, 170
Cameron, David, 251–2
Canada, 174, 177, 182, 251
  gender parity in, 254
Centers for Disease Control and Prevention, US, xvi, 33–4, 123
child soldiers, 102–3, 112, 121, 169, 261
  aid groups for, 120, 125–6
  appetitive aggression experienced by, 105–6
  as crime against humanity, 167
  recruitment/initiation of, 104, 105, 106–8, 167
China, 33, 119, 168, 250–1
  rapes in, 109, 199
Cishambo, Marcellin, 272
City of Joy, Bukavu, Congo, 92–8, 127, 160
Clinton, Bill, 154
Clinton Foundation, 152, 154
colleges, sexual assaults at, 124–5
Colombia peace talks, 256–7
colonialism, xiii, 3–17, 40, 54–5, 118–9
"comfort women," 197–203, 205
Community of Pentecostal Churches, Central Africa, 44, 85
Congo (Democratic Republic of the Congo). *See also* criminal justice system; rape/sexual violence
  "brain drain" in, 40–2
  colonialism in, xiii, 3–17, 40, 54–5, 118–9
  conflict casualties in, xiii, 170

Congo War, First, in, 48–57,
    75–6, 106–7, 110–3, 147,
    170–3, 208, 271
Congo War, Second, in, 57–83,
    106–7, 110–7, 135, 147–50,
    170–3, 208
corporal punishment in, 227–8
corruption in, 40, 85–6, 114–20,
    136–7, 146, 150–4, 158–62,
    164–5, 171, 188, 258–61
criminal justice system of,
    156–74, 275, 277
domestic violence in, 227, 228
economy of, 14–5, 26, 40, 97,
    99, 113–20, 146, 163, 173,
    208, 260
gender hierarchy in, 212–26,
    242–4
geographical characteristics of,
    8–10, 43, 113, 188
independence of, 12–3, 18–9
infrastructure of, 84–5, 119,
    136, 188, 258, 260
literacy levels in, 74–5
Mai-Mai militias in, 76–83,
    104–8, 111–6, 120–1, 129–32,
    150, 163–5, 187–93, 270
maternal health care in, 2, 8,
    25–7, 31–43, 56–7, 225
military of, 111–2, 127–32,
    161–5, 168
mineral industry in, 113–20,
    146, 163, 173, 208, 260
rape acknowledgment/
    reparations by, 137, 147,
    151–4, 161, 165, 172, 187–93,
    197, 209, 257–60, 269
Simba rebellion in, 162
Congo Free State (now Democratic
    Republic of Congo), 4, 118
Congolese military, 168
    courts, 127–32, 161–5
    rebels absorbed into, 111–2, 128
Conrad, Joseph, 59
consent, 179–80, 230–1
coronavirus pandemic, 41, 223,
    229, 253
corporal punishment, 227–8

corporate gender equity, 255
Cosby, Bill, 175
Council on Foreign Relations, 256
crime(s) against humanity, 170, 172
    child soldier recruitment as, 167
    rape as, 161–8, 171
criminal justice system. See also
    law enforcement; legislation,
    rape; prosecution of rape
    Congolese military and,
        127–32, 161–5
    corruption in, 158–62, 164–5,
        171
    international humanitarian
        law's role in, 161–74, 186
    Judicial Clinic, Panzi Hospital,
        and, 160–4
    war crimes/crimes against
        humanity in, 161–74, 186,
        208, 249–50, 252, 260–1
Crown Prosecution Service (UK),
    175

David (engineer), 49–50
Delivering Through Diversity
    study, 255
Democratic Forces for the
    Liberation of Rwanda
    (FDLR), 76–7, 89, 111, 130
Democratic Republic of the Congo.
    See Congo
Deneuve, Catherine, 140–1
Deschryver, Christine, 90–5, 279
Detroit, Michigan, 183–4
Dodd-Frank Act, US, 117
Dohuk refugee camp, Iraq,
    239–41
domestic violence, 227, 228, 275
Dovgan, Iryna, 141–2

Eastern Congo Initiative, 160
Egeland, Jan, 133–4, 136, 154
elders, leadership by, 244–9,
    275–6
EngenderHealth, 84
Ensler, Eve. See V

Epike (medical assistant), 30
Equality Now, 180
Equal Protection Clause,
    Fourteenth Amendment
    (US), 217
Equal Rights Amendment (ERA),
    217–8
ERA Coalition, 218
Esther (nurse), 91
Estonia, parental leave in, 35
ethnic cleansing, 108–10, 115
European Union
    Agency for Fundamental
        Rights, 174
    funding by, 84, 135, 209, 261
    Sakharov Prize by, 86
    women representatives of,
        253–4

false allegations of rape, 178
FARC, 256
FDLR. See Democratic Forces for
    the Liberation of Rwanda
female genital cutting, 245
feticide, female, 215
First Congo War (1996–1997), 48,
    52–54, 56–7, 112
    child soldiers in, 106–7
    Lemera Hospital attack in,
        49–51, 55, 147, 171, 208, 271
    Mapping Report on, 170–3,
        208
    massacres in, 50, 75–6, 271
    rapes in, 110–1, 147
    resource plundering in, 113
Fistula Foundation, 84
fistulas, 27, 36, 97, 148
    rapes resulting in, 62, 71, 72,
        77–81, 89
    treatment history of, 79–80
Fonda, Jane, 234
Foreign Policy, 161
Fragmentos (art installation),
    256–7
France, 123, 175, 223, 227
    gender parity in, 254, 255
    rape resolutions by, 209, 251

G-7 summits, 217, 252
General Social Survey on
    Victimization in Canada, 174
genocide, 118, 167
    in the Holocaust, 194–7
    rape as, 166, 250
    in Rwanda, 46–8, 56, 76, 108,
        110, 113, 170–2
Georgieva, Kristalina, 223
Germany, 41, 209, 223, 253, 261
    domestic violence in, 227
    Nazi, 108, 165–6, 194–7
Global and Inclusive Agreement,
    2002 (Congo), 135
Global Citizen Award, 152, 154
Global Gender Gap Report, 254
Global Initiative to End All
    Corporal Punishment of
    Children, 228
Global Media Monitoring Project,
    194
Global Study on Homicide, 143
Global Summit to End Sexual
    Violence in Conflict, 251
Global Witness, 119
Goddard, Marty, 183
Guevara, Che, 54
Guinea, 209, 245

Habyarimana, Juvénal, 47
Hague, William, 155, 251–2
Hamlin, Catherine, 79
Hamlin, Reginald, 79
Harvard University, 125
Haugstvedt, Svein, 24, 28–9, 42
Haya Bint al-Hussein, (princess of
    Jordan), 136
Hāzners, Vilis, 194
HEAL Africa, Congo, 62
health care
    "brain drain" in, 40–2
    maternal, 2, 8, 25–7, 31–43,
        56–7, 225
Hedgepeth, Sonja, 195–7
Heroinat statue, 204
historians, gender bias by,
    194–209, 275

HIV, xii, 89–90, 250, 277
Hochschild, Adam, 118
Hollaback!, 139
the Holocaust, rapes in, 194–7
Home Office (UK), 178
honor crimes/killings, 71, 143–4
Human Rights Watch, 132–3
Hurricane Katrina, 122–3, 234
Hutu people, 46—54, 58–9, 75,
    108, 110, 113, 166, 172.
    See also Rwanda
    FDLR of, 76–7, 89, 111, 130

ICC. *See* International Criminal
    Court
Idjwi, Congo, 269–75
India, 223
    rapes in, 144–5, 180
    WW II rapes by, 202–3
International Committee of the
    Red Cross, 47
International Criminal Court
    (ICC), 166–7, 174, 252, 261
    budget for, 173
    opposition to, 168–9
International Criminal Tribunal for
    Rwanda, 47, 166, 170–1, 249
    expansion to Congo, 172
International Criminal Tribunal
    for the former Yugoslavia,
    166, 170, 249
international humanitarian law
    implementation of, 166–74, 186
    rape's classification in, 161–8,
    171
International Labor Organization,
    34
International Rescue Committee,
    170
Inter-Parliamentary Union, 254
In the Body of the World
    (Ensler/V), 94
Iraq, rapes in, 110, 115, 180, 186,
    205, 209, 236–42, 244, 277
ISIS (Islamic State), rape by, 115,
    123, 205, 210, 237–42, 244
It's On Us initiative, 139

Jahjaga, Atifete, 204
Janjaweed militia, Sudan, 137
Japan, 209
    war rapes by, 109, 165–6,
    197–203, 205
Jeanne (rape survivor), 92–3, 98,
    138, 205, 277
Jeshi la Yesu group, 162
Jolie, Angelina, 251
Joseph (Mukwege employee),
    266–8
Journal of Communication, 233

Kabarebe, James, 57
Kabila, Joseph, 111, 119, 135–6,
    261
    Panzi Hospital visit by, 257–60
    rape acknowledgment and,
    137, 147, 151–3, 161, 172,
    192–3, 197, 257–60, 269
Kabila, Laurent-Désiré, 50, 54,
    57–8, 76, 107, 111, 135
Kaboyi (Denis's father-in-law),
    36–7, 53–4
Kabungulu, Pascal, 55
Kagame, Paul, 46, 48, 114, 172,
    261
Kang Kyung-wha, 189
Katanga, Germain, 167
Katuku militia, 104–8, 120–1
Kavumu, Congo, 156–63, 167,
    186, 208, 270
Kaziba, Congo, 2, 13–8, 53, 171
Kelly, R., 175
Kenya, 54–5
Khmer Rouge, 170
Kim Bok-dong, 198–202, 205
Kim Hak-sun, 200
King Leopold's Ghost (Hochschild),
    118
Kinshasa, Congo, 9, 24, 54, 114,
    128, 258
    clinic in, 210–1, 277
Kokodikoko (warlord), 163–4, 165
Kosovo, war rapes in, 203–5
Krasniqi-Goodman, Vasfije, 203–5
Kulungu, Thérèse, 160

The Last Girl (Murad), 237
law enforcement. *See also*
    criminal justice system;
    prosecution of rape
  civil, 156–61, 165, 173–4
  corruption in, 158–62, 164–5,
    171
  evidence-gathering by, 181–4
  international, 47, 165–74, 186,
    196, 249, 252, 261
  military, 127–32, 161–5
  statutes of limitation in, 184–5
  training of, 181–4
leadership
  deficient, 257–62
  by elders, 244–9, 275–6
  in peace processes, 250, 256–7
  religious, 236, 241–4, 275–6
  by UN/global institutions,
    249–52, 261
  by women, 252–7, 278
Lebel, Jean, 268–9
legislation, rape, xvi–xvii, 178
  on consent, 179, 180
  gender bias in, 217, 219
  implementation of, 180–4
Lemera Hospital, Congo, 62
  attack on, 49–51, 55, 147, 171,
    208, 271
  Mukwege as medical director
    of, 42–3, 46–51, 55, 62, 147,
    171, 208
  Mukwege as student doctor at,
    23–4, 26–37, 39
Leopold II, (king of Belgium), 4,
    12, 14, 16, 118
Leo XIII, Pope, 4
Lewis, Stephen, xii
LGBTQ, 125, 251
Lirzin, Roger Le, 42
Löfven, Stefan, 251
Loyola University, 122
Lubanga, Thomas, 167
Lumumba, Patrice, 12–3, 119

M23. *See* National Congress for
    the Defense of the People

Macron, Emmanuel, 217, 251
Magambo (medic), 269
Mai-Mai (Congolese militias),
    76–83, 104–8, 111–6, 120–1,
    129–32, 150, 163–5, 187–93,
    270
Maison Dorcas, Bukavu, Congo,
    97, 149, 160
Mapping Report (UN), 170–3,
    208
marital rape, 178, 180
Maroney, McKayla, 143
Martius, Heinrich, 80
maternal health care, 37–41
  in Congo, 2, 8, 25–7, 31–6,
    42–3, 56–7, 225
  maternal death rates and, 2, 8,
    32–3, 42
  physical labor's impact on, 34,
    42, 225
McKinsey & Company, 255
Médecins Sans Frontières (MSF;
    Doctors Without Borders),
    78, 81–3
media, 161, 275
  gender bias in, 186, 193–6
men. *See also* positive masculinity
  corporal punishment and,
    227–8
  cultural expectations and,
    25–6, 29–32, 42, 212–6,
    219–26
  domestic violence by, 227, 228
  economic power of, 15, 26, 223
  education of, 138, 219–22
  gender hierarchy and, 212–26,
    242–4
  pay gap and, 218–9
  positive masculinity by, xvii,
    31–2, 212–35, 245–9
  rape of, 66–7
  role models for, 226–35
  sex discussions by, 230–3
Merkel, Angela, 209, 252–3
#MeToo movement, xvi, 139–41,
    143, 174–5, 200, 209, 218,
    232, 274
Miller, Chanel, 177

mineral industry, 118
  exploitation of, 113–7, 119–20,
    146, 163, 173, 208, 260
  rape's tie to, 113–6
Ministry of Health, Congo, 227
Mission Aviation Fellowship, 52
Mobutu, Joseph, 24, 40, 42,
    48–9, 51, 54, 57–8, 119, 162
MONUC (United Nations
    Organization Mission in the
    Democratic Republic of the
    Congo), 132–3, 135, 147,
    157, 163, 172–3, 190, 263,
    266, 272, 276
Moreno-Ocampo, Luis, 167
Mukanire, Tatiana, 99–100, 112,
    205, 277
Mukwege, Denis
  assassination attempts on, 147,
    155, 264–74
  awards/prizes received by, 86,
    117, 148, 152, 154, 205–11,
    237, 276
  birth/childhood of, 1–8, 12–4,
    18–22, 212–4
  City of Joy and, 92–5, 127, 160
  education of, 19, 23–5, 36–40,
    148
  escape from Bukavu by, 51–5,
    267–74
  intimidation of, 146–7, 151–5,
    165, 257, 264, 267
  Lemera practice by, 23–4, 26–37,
    39, 42–3, 46–51, 55, 62
  Maison Dorcas and, 97, 149,
    160
  marriage of, 36–7
  medical specialties of, 8,
    36–40, 65–6
  Panzi Hospital practice by,
    44–8, 55–73, 74–100,
    127–34, 147–50, 156–7, 160,
    187, 206–7, 210–1, 257–60,
    263–78
  refugee work by, 54–5, 113
  SEMA network and, 99, 203
  UN speeches by, 86–7, 134–8,
    146, 147, 151–5, 267

Mukwege, Denise, 146, 153,
    266–71
Mukwege, Elizabeth, 214–6
Mukwege, Lina, 146, 153, 266–71
Mukwege, Madeleine, 38, 42–3,
    51–5, 146, 153–4, 208, 212,
    266–72
  career of, 40, 63
  marriage of, 36–7
Mukwege, Mr. (Denis's father),
    1, 212
  death of, 215
  positive masculinity and, 226,
    229
  profession of, 4–5, 11, 17–22, 23
Mukwege, Ms. (Denis's mother),
    xiv, 17–8, 22, 272
  gender bias and, 212–4, 226,
    229
Mukwege, Roda, 214–6
Mungo (radiologist), 45
Murad, Nadia, 205–7, 209, 237–40
Mutebusi, Jules, 99
mutual solidarity organizations
    (MUSOs), 97, 99, 277
Mwenga, Congo, 171
Myanmar, 110, 186, 206, 210
My Name Is Kim Bok Dong
    (documentary), 203

Nairobi, Kenya, 54–5, 113
Nangini, Cathy, 115
Nassar, Larry, 143
National Congress for the Defense
    of the People (M23), 114,
    251, 261
National Health Service, UK, 41
National Sexual Violence
    Resource Center, US, 122,
    178
Native Americans, 33–4
Nazi Germany
  rapes by, 108, 165–6, 194–7
  war trials, 165–6, 196
NDAs. See non-disclosure
    agreements
Neuwirth, Jessica, 189, 218

The New York Times, 175, 183
New York University, 87
Nigeria, 206, 210
Nkunda, Laurent, 99, 112, 168
Nobel Peace Prize, 86, 117,
    205–11, 237, 276
non-disclosure agreements
    (NDAs), 142–3
Norway, 15–6, 141, 253, 255
Ntaganda, Bosco, 167–8, 261
Ntaryamira, Cyprien, 47
Nuremburg trials, 165–6, 196

Obama, Barack, 139, 251, 261
Olof Palme Prize, 148
Organisation for Economic
    Co-operation and
    Development (OECD), 34,
    117, 218, 223, 227, 254–5

Panzi Foundation, 86
    City of Joy and, 92–5, 127, 160
    Judicial Clinic of, 160–4
    Maison Dorcas and, 97, 149,
        160
Panzi Hospital, Bukavu, Congo,
    272–8
    construction of, 44–6, 55–8,
        83–4
    evidence gathering at, 181
    funding of, 83–6
    infrastructure systems of, 84–6
    Judicial Clinic of, 160–4
    psychological support team at,
        64–5, 72, 82, 92–8, 138, 149,
        181–2, 240, 256
    rape victims at, 59–73, 76–83,
        88–92, 98–9, 127–34, 138,
        146, 148–50, 156–63, 169,
        173, 181, 187, 190, 206–8,
        210, 257–60
parental leave, 34–5
parenting
    corporal punishment in, 227–8
    domestic/unpaid labor division
        and, 212–6

macho conditioning *vs.*
    positive masculinity in,
    228–35
    sex education in, 230–3
    women's advocacy via, xvii,
        275–6
Park Geun-hye, 201
pay gap, 218–9
peace process, gender parity in,
    250, 256–7
Physicians for Human Rights,
    160–1, 268
Pillay, Navi, 166, 171
Planned Parenthood, 231
PLOS Medicine, 115
PL+US (Paid Leave for the United
    States), 35
politics, gender parity in, 252–5,
    278
polygamy, 26, 215
pornography, 232–3
positive masculinity, xvii, 31–2
    via Badilika program, 222–6,
        245–9
    gender hierarchy and, 212–26,
        242–4
    macho/toxic conditioning *vs.*,
        228–35
    role models for, 226–35
    sex education aiding, 230–2
Power, Samantha, 205
prenatal care, 25, 27, 33, 39, 42–3
prosecution of rape, xvi, 156–7,
    179, 203–4, 274–5. *See also*
    criminal justice system; law
    enforcement; legislation, rape
    corruption and, 158–62, 164–5
    evidence-gathering for, 181–4
    false allegations and, 178
    first responder training and,
        181–4
    by international courts/laws,
        47, 165–74, 186, 196, 249,
        252, 261
    Mapping Report and, 170–3, 208
    in marriages, 178, 180
    presumption of innocence/
        guilt in, 180–1

statute of limitations on, 184–5
systematic bias in, 176–8,
    185–6
as war crime, 161–8, 171,
    249–50, 260
in Western countries, 174–7
Putin, Vladimir, 202

Rally for Congolese Democracy
    (RCD), 57, 111
Rape, Abuse & Incest National
    Network (RAINN), 174–5
rape crisis centers, 182
rape kits, 183–4
rape motivation
    economic profit as, 110, 113–7,
        146, 171, 208
    ethnic cleansing as, 108–10, 115
    revenge/thrill as, 104–7, 109, 121
    terror campaigns as, 109–12, 115
rape, recognition of
    by Congo government, 137, 147,
        151–4, 161, 165, 172, 187–93,
        197, 209, 257–60, 269
    in media/historic
        documentation, 193–209,
        275
    via reparations, 189–93, 204,
        209–11, 256
    via storytelling, 90–1, 127–34,
        138–9, 154, 173, 191–2,
        198–200, 203–5
    in WW II, 108–9, 194–203, 205
rape/sexual violence. See also
        advocacy, women's rights
    AIDS/HIV resulting from,
        89–90, 277
    by Allied forces, 109, 202–3
    awareness campaigns on, 83,
        127, 139–41, 143, 274
    in Bosnia and Herzegovina,
        109–10, 115, 166, 197, 203–5
    in colleges, 124–5
    consent discussions and,
        179–80, 230–1
    culture of, 123–5
    false allegations of, 178

fistulas resulting from, 62, 71,
    72, 77–81, 89
in former Yugoslavia, 109–10,
    115, 166, 197, 203–5
honor killings associated with,
    71, 143–4
investigation/prosecution of,
    xvi, 47, 156–86, 196, 203–4,
    208, 249–50, 260–1, 274–5
by Islamic extremists, 115,
    123, 205, 210, 237–42, 244
by Japan, 109, 165–6, 197–203,
    205
male victims of, 66–7
marital, 178, 180
media/historic recognition of,
    193–209, 275
in Myanmar, 118, 186, 206,
    210
in natural disasters, 122–3, 234
by Nazi Germany, 108, 165–6,
    194–7
pregnancies resulting from, 97,
    149–50
propensity for, 59–60
psychological support post-,
    64–5, 72, 82, 92–8, 138,
    149, 160, 181–2, 240–1, 256,
    274–5
shame/guilt associated with,
    65, 82–3, 126, 132, 143,
    145–6, 154, 193, 195, 274
by Soviet forces, 108–9, 202
statistics on, xvi, 62, 123, 174
stigma associated with, 68,
    70–2, 82–3, 126, 195, 274–5
trauma associated with, 61–7,
    70–1, 81–3, 89–100, 149,
    157, 177, 181–2, 204, 240,
    257, 275
victim blaming in, 71–2, 177,
    275
victim reparations for, 189–93,
    204, 209–11, 256
virginity tests post-, 176–8
as war crime/crime against
    humanity, 161–8, 171,
    249–50, 260

Ravensbrück concentration camp, Germany, 195
Rehn, Elizabeth, 189
religion
  evangelism in, 3–9, 15–9
  gender bias in, 236, 241–4, 249
Remember the Women Institute, 194
Republic of Zaire, 40. *See also* Congo
Rohingya women, 210
Roland (medic), 52
Ronald Feldman Gallery, New York City, 197
Rousseff, Dilma, 209
Russia, 202, 249–51. *See also* Soviet Union
Rwanda, 14, 23, 43, 271
  Congo resource pillaging by, 113–7, 119, 163, 173
  Congo Wars and, 106–7, 147–50, 170–3
  genocide in/by, 46–8, 56, 76, 108, 110, 113, 170–2
  International Criminal Tribunal for, 47, 166, 170–2, 249
  Mapping Report and, 171–3
  post-Congo War militias of, 99, 107, 114, 130, 133–5, 148–50, 167–8, 191, 251, 261, 267
  rape as weapon of war in, 108–11, 115, 166, 197, 249–50
  US and UK support to, 135, 148, 172, 261
Rwandan Patriotic Front, 48

Saidel, Rochelle G., 194–7
Sakharov Prize, 86
Salcedo, Doris, 256–7
Sanguinetti, Michael, 71–2
Santos, Juan Manuel, 256
Savanta ComRes, 232
Schiappa, Marlène, 223
Scott, Bart, 234
Second Congo War (1998–2003), 112, 135
  child soldiers in, 106–7

Mapping Report on, 170–3, 208
origins of, 57–8
rapes in, 59–73, 74–83, 110–1, 147–50
resource plundering in, 113–7
SEMA network, 99, 203
Sengar, Kuldeep Singh, 144–5
Serbia, war rapes by, 109–10, 115, 166, 197, 203–5
Sexual Violence Against Jewish Women During the Holocaust (Saidel/Hedgepeth), 195
Shabunda, Congo, 129–32, 154, 187–93, 209, 211
Sierra Leone, 109
  Special Court for, 170
Simba rebellion, Congo, 162
Sims, James Marion, 79–80
slaves, 3, 14
  medical experimentation on, 80
  sex, 77–8, 89, 108, 168, 238
Slutwalk movement, 72, 274
South Africa, 169, 223
South Korea, 209
  "comfort women" of, 197–203, 205
Soviet Union, 13, 119. *See also* Russia
  WW II rapes by, 108–9, 202
statute of limitations, 184–5
Stop Rape Now, 139
Sudan, rapes in, 137, 186
Sweden, 7, 41, 148, 223, 261
  consent laws in, 179
  evangelists from, 18–9, 23, 83–4
  feminist foreign policy of, 251
  gender parity in, 254
Swedish International Development Cooperation Agency, 83
Syria, rapes in, 115, 186, 206

Take Back the Night, 139
Taylor, Charles, 170
30% Club, 255
Time's Up, 139

Tokyo trials, WW II, 165–6
TRIAL International, 160
Trudeau, Justin, 251
Trump, Donald, 168, 218, 229,
    232, 250
Tshisekedi, Félix, 261
Turner, Brock, 177, 231
Tutsi people, 46—54, 58–9, 75–7,
    108, 110–1, 113, 166, 168.
    See also Rwanda
    M23 rebel group of, 114, 251,
    261
Twain, Mark, 118

Uganda, 14, 46–7, 167, 169
    Congo Wars and, 50, 57–8,
    106–7, 113–7, 147, 170
    resource pillaging by, 113–7
Ukraine, 141–2
UNESCO, 75
UNICEF, 57–8, 227
    City of Joy funding by, 92
United Arab Emirates (UAE),
    116–7
United Kingdom (UK), 41, 84,
    118, 223, 233
    domestic violence in, 227
    rape prosecutions in, 175, 182
    rape resolutions by, 209,
    251–2, 261
    rape statistics in, 123
    Rwanda support by, 135, 148,
    172, 261
    WW II rapes by, 109, 202–3
United Nations (UN), 57–8, 75, 92,
    99, 113, 116, 178, 227, 269
    Human Rights Council, 204
    Human Rights Monitoring
    Mission, 141
    Millennium Development
    Goals of, 33
    Mukwege speeches to, 86–7,
    134–8, 146, 147, 151–5, 267
    Office of the Special
    Representative of the
    Secretary-General on Sexual
    Violence in Conflict, 150, 250
    Office of the UN High
    Commissioner for Human
    Rights, 170–3, 189, 209
    Office on Drugs and Crime,
    123, 143
    peacekeeping forces, xii–xiii,
    132–3, 135, 147, 157, 163,
    172–3, 190, 263, 266, 272, 276
    Population Fund, 143
    Prize in the Field of Human
    Rights, 148
    rape resolutions by, 209,
    249–51
    Security Council, 205, 249–51
United States (US), 33–5, 41, 119,
    168, 223
    conflict minerals and, 117, 208
    Congo funding/support by, 84,
    261
    domestic violence in, 227
    rape prosecutions in, 174, 177,
    182
    rape resolutions by, 251, 261
    rape/sexual assault by military
    of, 60, 109, 124, 202–3
    rape statistics in, xvi, 123,
    124–5
    Rwanda support by, 135, 148,
    172, 261
United States Agency for
    International Development,
    84
University of Ghent, Belgium, 148
University of Michigan, 125
UN Women, 178
USA Gymnastics, 143
US Constitution, 217
US Department of Defense, 124
US Department of Labor, 34
US House of Representatives, 204
US Marine Corps, 124
US Supreme Court, 217

V (formerly Eve Ensler), 87–95,
    98, 127, 139, 206, 234
The Vagina Monologues (play),
    87–8, 234

V-Day organization, 92–5, 234
Veikko (surgeon), 45
victim blaming, 71–2, 177, 275
Vietnam War, rapes in, 60, 109
VIOLATED exhibition, 197
virginity tests, 176–8

Wakubenga (rape survivor),
    149–50, 152, 154, 277
Wallström, Margot, 150, 153–4
Wamuzila (rape survivor), 74–83,
    87, 88–94, 96–9, 187
War and Women's Human Rights
    Museum, Seoul, South
    Korea, 198
war crime(s)
    ICC's role in prosecuting,
        166–9, 173–4, 252, 261
    international humanitarian law
        on, 161–74, 186
    Mapping Report on, 170–3, 208
    prosecution, in Congo, of,
        161–4, 167–70
    rape's classification as, 161–8,
        171, 249–50, 260
Warega people, 224–6, 245–9
The War Within the War, 133
Washington, Kerry, 234
The Washington Post, 201
Weinstein, Harvey, 140, 142, 175,
    186
Williams, Whitney, 160
Witula (rape survivor), 129–32,
    154, 187, 276
Wolfe, Lauren, 161
women. *See also* advocacy,
    women's rights; maternal
    health care; rape/sexual
    violence
    advocacy by, xii–xiii, xvi–xvii,
        87–100, 252–7, 269–75
    corporal punishment and, 227–8
    cultural expectations of, 25–6,
        29–32, 42

discriminatory laws against,
    217, 219
domestic bias/labor division
    and, 212–6, 219, 222–6, 275
domestic violence against, 227,
    228, 275
economic power of, 15, 26, 97,
    99, 223, 254
education/literacy of, 74–5,
    219–22, 254
gender hierarchy and, 212–26,
    242–4
genital cutting and, 245
leadership by, 252–7, 278
maternal health care for, 2, 8,
    25–7, 31–43, 56–7, 225
murder statistics on, 143
pay gap for, 218–9
political parity for, 252–5, 278
religious gender bias and,
    241–4, 249
sex education as benefit to,
    230–3
valuation of, xvii, 70–3, 101,
    104–5, 120–6, 169, 180, 186,
    212–35, 242
World Economic Forum, 219, 254
World Health Organization
    (WHO), 27, 41, 123
World War I (WW I), 119
World War II (WW II), xiii, 119
    rape's occurrence in, 108–9,
        194–203, 205
    war trials for, 165–6

Yale University, 125, 174
Yazda organization, 237–41
Yazidi women, 205, 237–42, 244,
    277
Yugoslavia, former
    International Criminal Tribunal
        for, 166, 170, 249
    rapes in, 109–10, 115, 166,
        197, 203–5

ABOUT THE AUTHOR

Dr. Denis Mukwege was born in the Belgian Congo in 1955. As a child and young man, he was a firsthand witness to racial prejudices, as well as to the economic and moral decay of the Democratic Republic of the Congo under dictatorship. Now a renowned gynecological surgeon, he is recognized as the world's leading expert on treating rape injuries, and his holistic approach to healing has inspired other initiatives around the world. In 2014 he was invited to the White House by President Barack Obama and, in Europe, he was awarded the prestigious Sakharov Prize, earning him major public recognition for the first time. In 2018, he was awarded the Nobel Peace Prize along with Yazidi human rights activist and sexual violence survivor Nadia Murad.